Two-Dimensional Echocardiography in Congenital Heart Disease

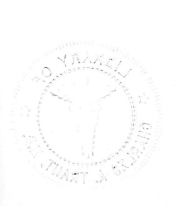

Two-Dimensional Echocardiography in Congenital Heart Disease

Norman H. Silverman, M.D.
Associate Professor of Pediatrics and Radiology (Cardiology)
Department of Pediatrics
University of California, San Francisco
San Francisco, California

A. Rebecca Snider, M.D.
Assistant Professor of Pediatrics (Cardiology)
Department of Pediatrics
University of California, San Francisco
San Francisco, California

APPLETON-CENTURY-CROFTS/Norwalk, Connecticut

Prentice-Hall International, Inc., London
Prentice-Hall of Australia, Pty. Ltd., Sydney
Prentice-Hall of India Private Limited, New Delhi
Prentice-Hall of Japan, Inc., Tokyo
Prentice-Hall of Southeast Asia (Pte.) Ltd., Singapore
Whitehall Books Ltd., Wellington, New Zealand

Library of Congress Cataloging in Publication Data

Silverman, Norman H.
    Two-dimensional echocardiography in congenital heart disease.

    Includes index.
    1. Ultrasonic cardiography. 2. Pediatric cardiology–Diagnosis.
3. Heart–Abnormalities–Diagnosis. I. Snider, Arleen Rebecca.
II. Title III. Title: 2-dimensional echocardiography in congenital heart disease.
RJ423.5.U46S54   618.92'1207543   81-20612
ISBN 0-8385-9058-6   AACR2

Cover and text design: Lucinda C. Carbuto
Production Editor: George Hachtel

PRINTED IN THE UNITED STATES OF AMERICA

To our parents—
Sim and Jean Silverman, Irma and Gifford
Snider—who led us into academic pursuits.

To our spouses and children—
Heather, Gina, Adam, and Claire
Silverman and Rick Hahn for their love,
endurance, and support.

Contents

Preface

Physicians, ultrasound technicians, and students who are involved in the care of patients with congenital heart disease need a comprehensive reference on two-dimensional echocardiography. With recent advances in medical and surgical therapy, increasingly more patients with congenital heart disease are surviving into adulthood. The two-dimensional echocardiogram is a valuable technique for the initial evaluation of these patients and for their serial assessment postoperatively.

The aim of this book is to provide a visual and descriptive reference for both the normal and abnormal cardiac anatomy encountered during two-dimensional echocardiography in patients with congenital heart disease. This volume is intended to be read after the acquisition of basic skills and knowledge in echocardiography and cardiology. We have avoided lengthy descriptions of the clinical presentation and management of the disorders and have provided only the information which is germane to the echocardiogram itself. We have also attempted to describe how the technique of two-dimensional echocardiography can be integrated into the overall clinical evaluation.

The data for this volume was collected over a five year period from two-dimensional echocardiographic studies in over 6000 patients admitted to the University of California at San Francisco. The data was validated by information obtained at cardiac catheterization, surgery, or autopsy.

The emphasis of this text is on the figures themselves which were chosen to provide an atlas of normal and abnormal cardiac anatomy. The display of the two-dimensional echocardiogram is dynamic and, by necessity, we have used photographs derived from stop-frame images. Some of the information obtained in the real-time recording from integration by the human eye and brain is lost in the stop-frame images. This fact should be borne in mind when examining some of the figures presented in this book.

Two-dimensional echocardiography, while highly developed, is still a rapidly growing technique. Although this text is as current as possible, the final chapters remain to be written.

Acknowledgments

We would like to express our deepest appreciation to Dr. Abraham Rudolph. His teaching, support, and encouragement led to the development of the pediatric echocardiography laboratory. Through his influence, we have worked in a rich environment which stimulates the growth of new ideas. We are also thankful for the support of our colleagues Drs. Saul Robinson, Paul Stanger, Michael Heymann, Julien Hoffman, Harold Tarnoff, Marvin Auerback and the many other physicians who have referred patients to us. We are especially grateful to Dr. Nelson Schiller who encouraged us in our early echo experiences and continues to exchange new ideas and information with us.

Our individual backgrounds and experiences have been different. One of us (N.H.S.) received early training in South Africa under the guidance of Drs. Solomon Levin, John Barlow, Jack Wolfsdorf, and John Hansen, N.H.S. is grateful for the association with Drs. Richard Popp and James French at Stanford University.

A.R.S. would like to thank Dr. L.H.S. van Mierop whose teachings have provided her with a basis for understanding cross-sectional echocardiography in congenital heart disease. A.R.S. is also grateful for education received in South Carolina from Drs. Arno Hohn, Donald Riopel, Ashby Taylor, and Hazel Webb, and in Philadelphia from Drs. Sidney Friedman and William Rashkind.

A special note of thanks goes to Ms. Debra Chodkowski who single-handedly typed, collated, and edited this manuscript. A special acknowledgment goes to the late Mr. William Bunker who skillfully prepared all of the photographic material for this book.

We are indebted to Dr. Tom Risser for the clarity and simplicity of his chapter on physics and instrumentation.

Foreword

Echocardiography, or ultrasonic cardiography, was not generally considered to be a useful research or diagnostic aid until the early 1970s. Perhaps no diagnostic procedure has gained more rapid and widespread application in medicine. Over the past ten years echocardiography has been used for assessing cardiac valve motion and function as well as ventricular wall motion and myocardial function, and for identification of cardiac abnormalities. During the early phases of development the technique had limited applicability in infants and children with congenital heart disease because the M-mode display provided a restricted view of a pencil-like probe through the heart. The development of two-dimensional real-time echocardiography has made it an almost essential tool in detailed evaluation of the patient with congenital heart disease. The information obtained by echocardiography complements that derived from cardiac catheterization and angiocardiography. Angiography defines the cavities of the heart and great vessels as well as the blood flow patterns. It is not ideal, however, for defining cardiac valve motion and function or ventricular wall thickness and movement. Two-dimensional real-time echocardiography is also capable of defining the cardiac chambers and great vessels and attachments, but has the advantages of demonstrating thickness of ventricular walls, wall motion and, especially, in showing valve action. With recent application of contrast echocardiography, course of blood flow within the heart can also be examined.

A major advantage of echocardiography is that the technique is not invasive. This has made it especially useful as a screening diagnostic tool in the newborn infant with cardiorespiratory distress and suspected heart disease. It has greatly reduced the frequency with which cardiac catheterization and angiography are required in sick infants to exclude the possible presence of a remedial cardiac lesion.

In this treatise Drs. Silverman and Snider present the principles of two-dimensional echocardiography and explain its application in diagnosis of congenital heart disease with great clarity. They have a vast experience in the use of two-dimensional echocardiography in diagnosis of complex congenital anomalies, and have pioneered many of the techniques. The material they have compiled demonstrates the remarkable precision that can be achieved in defining abnormal cardiac structure and function. The meticulous attention to photographic procedures and accompanying diagrams makes the presentation understandable even to those uninitiated in echocardiographic technics. This volume depicts the current achievements, but we can look forward to dramatic improvements in ultrasound resolution of cardiac and vascular structures with even better definition than is currently possible. Also, the application of Doppler flow analysis will undoubtedly extend the usefulness of ultrasound in cardiac diagnosis.

Abraham M. Rudolph, MD

Two-Dimensional Echocardiography in Congenital Heart Disease

CHAPTER 1

Two-Dimensional Echocardiographic Systems: Physics and Instrumentation

Thomas B. Risser

Most textbooks on the application of ultrasonic imaging to medical diagnosis begin with a lengthy discussion of the physical principles of ultrasound. The usual reason given for this approach is that the user of an instrument must master its principles of operation in order to use it properly. The authors of the present text, however, do not share this view. Our modern electronic society is filled with instruments whose workings are not understood by average users. Diagnostic ultrasound equipment is especially complex and cannot be explained adequately in a textbook on medical technique. However, there are certain points the users should know in order to have an idea of the choices that are open to them in the purchase and use of ultrasonic scanners. We will present the most important facts without too much discussion of the underlying physics. The reference at the end of this chapter is for those readers wishing a more detailed description.[1]

PULSE-ECHO ULTRASOUND INSTRUMENTS

The ultrasonic waves used in diagnostic instruments are generated by piezoelectric crystals. Such crystals have an atomic structure that causes them to vibrate when an electrical signal is applied and, conversely, to emit an electrical signal when they are made to vibrate. To generate the ultrasonic beam that will enter the patient, a piezoelectric crystal or transducer is pulsed electronically and made to vibrate at megaHertz frequencies, in most cases between 2.25 and 5.0 MHz. The crystal vibration is very short in duration, and induced vibrations travel outward as a pulse into the patient. This pulse is an ultrahigh frequency sound wave. Such sound waves behave like electromagnetic waves

1

in that they are reflected, refracted, dispersed, and attenuated. Dispersion and attenuation occur as the waves pass through any homogeneous medium. Reflection and refraction occur at boundaries between different media, for example at the boundary between the blood and myocardium. Normally, the reflection is small and most of the sound wave (i.e., the refracted part) continues further into the patient. Those reflected waves that return directly to the transducer cause it to vibrate and, therefore, emit an electrical signal. This signal is received by the electronics.

The diagnostic instrument contains "smart" electronics that "knows" (1) when the pulse was emitted, (2) when the echo returned, (3) how large the returning echo was, and (4) how fast sound travels in the human body. Thus, the electronics determines how deep in the body the echo was produced. The distance to the echo-producing boundary and the size of the echo are stored electronically until enough such echoes are received to form an image, which is then displayed on a screen (usually a video screen). This is the basic operation of diagnostic pulse-echo systems. The pulse-echo process can be done extremely quickly, as often as 4000 times per second scanning to a depth of 20 cm and even faster for shallower scanning.

SECTOR SCANNERS

At present, two-dimensional cardiac imaging is done almost exclusively with a special type of pulse-echo instrument called a sector scanner. Sector scanners now come in two forms: (1) electronic scanners (phased arrays) in which the ultrasonic beam is aimed electronically and (2) mechanical scanners in which the beam is aimed mechanically. Both types of scanners produce a pie-shaped or sector image. The beam is aimed by the instrument in one direction and pulsed. The electronics waits for and receives all echoes expected to return from the scanning depth chosen. Then the transducer is aimed in another direction and the process is repeated. The pattern of directions along which the pulse-echo data is collected is shown in Figure 1-1.

The sector scanner's "smart" electronics "knows" one fact more than the simplest pulse-echo instrument described above. It also "knows" what the beam direction is. Therefore, the sector scanner electronics "knows" and stores both the size of the echo and exactly where it came from (both direction and depth) to within the resolution of the beam. In a typical sector scanner, the sector angle will be 80 to 90 degrees; and, when scanning to a depth of 20 cm, there will be roughly 128 scan lines. The image will be obtained, stored, and displayed 30 times per second. Thus, the basic pulse-echo process will be repeated $30 \times 128 = 3840$ times per second. If the instrument only scanned to a 10-cm depth, the electronics would only have to wait half as long for the returning echoes. It could then repeat the basic pulse-echo process twice as often, meaning that the electronics could either produce 128 lines 60 times per second or 256 lines 30 times per second. Some instruments allow the user to make such a choice by a front panel switch or knob.

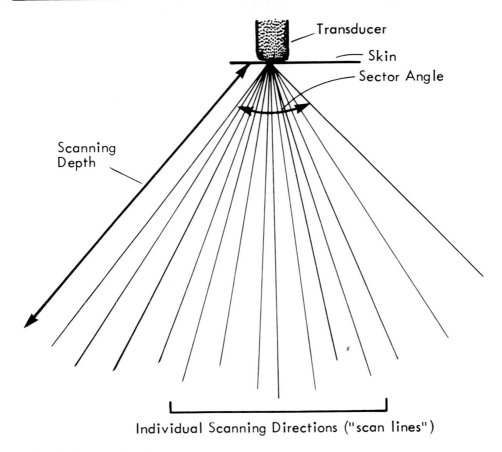

FIG. 1-1. *Sector scanning pattern.*

Before leaving the subject of the sector scanner's image pattern (Fig. 1-1), let us note one important fact that we will return to later in the discussion on digital data processing. The sector scanner electronics "thinks" that the returning echo has come along the chosen scan line. Actually, because the ultrasonic beam has a finite width (i.e., finite resolution as discussed below), the echo may really come from a point near, but not actually on, the scan line. However, the electronics "thinks" the echo was actually on the line and stores and displays the echo as if that were the case. Since the lines radiate outward from the point of transducer-patient contact, the displayed points making up the image in the far field are much less dense than those in the near field. Digital data processing can do something about this, thereby improving the far-field image.

Mechanical sector scanners are simpler conceptually than electronic sector scanners. A solid transducer, usually circular, is moved in an arc by purely mechanical means. Figure 1-2 shows the two principal techniques in use

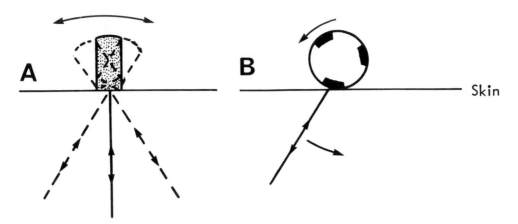

FIG. 1-2. *Types of mechanical sector scanners.* **A.** *Rocking transducer,* **B.** *spinning transducers.*

today. In the older technique (Fig. 1-2A), a single transducer element is rocked back and forth at the point of contact with the patient's skin. More recently, spinning transducers have been introduced (Fig. 1-2B). In this technique, one or more transducers are mounted on a small wheel that spins at constant velocity. One transducer transmits and receives through the scanning arc, and, as it finishes the desired arc, the next transducer on the wheel takes over, and so forth.

The electronic sector scanners, called phased arrays, operate on more complex principles. A single rectangular transducer is cut into a series of parallel strips, usually 32 in number, which then become a series of 32 small, narrow, and independent transducers. By controlling the exact time of activation (phase) of the individual transducer elements, the outgoing beam can be steered in any desired direction (Fig. 1-3A). The beam can also be focused in a given direction (Fig. 1-3B) if curvature is introduced into the phasing.

Each element in the phased array creates a cylindrical outgoing wave. As these waves move outward from the transducer, they merge together (i.e., interfere constructively) to form the beam. Once the sound waves are approximately 20 wavelengths (about 1 cm) away from the transducer, the sound beam is formed to the same degree it would have been had it come from a solid transducer (i.e., one not cut into strips). Therefore, when resolution is discussed below, the same general statements about beam dimension and divergence apply to both electronic and mechanical sector scanner beams. The electronic scanner beams come from a rectangular transducer, and the mechanical scanner beams come from a circular transducer. This means that they are slightly, but only slightly, different in spatial cross section. The principal differences are that the phased arrays can direct the beam at an angle to the transducer face and focus the beam electronically (i.e., without a lens),

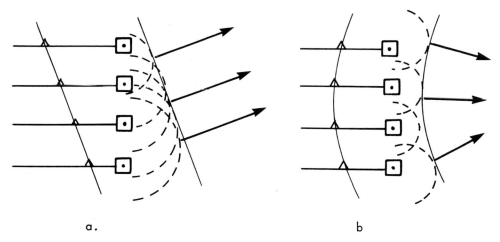

FIG. 1-3. *Beam formation from phased array.* **A.** *Unfocused,* **B.** *focused.*

whereas the mechanical sector scanners cannot. Otherwise, the properties of the outgoing beams are very similar.

Resolution

Resolution is one of the most important characteristics of a diagnostic ultra-sound instrument that determines the quality of the image. It is not, however, the only important characteristic, as we shall see below when penetrating power, sensitivity, image processing, and transducer size are discussed. Resolution is the ability of the system to distinguish between reflections from nearby objects. Resolution in depth, usually called axial resolution (i.e., along the direction of the beam), is quite different and much better than lateral resolution (i.e., perpendicular to the beam).

Depth resolution is determined by the length in space of the outgoing sound wave pulse and is remarkably uniform from one instrument to another. The average outgoing pulse is roughly 1.5 mm in length for a 3.0-MHz transducer, which translates to an axial resolution of roughly 1.5 mm. If there are two objects producing echoes, one directly behind the other, and they are more than 1.5 mm apart, then the returning echoes will be separate in time. The instrument's electronics will receive two distinct echoes, consequently recognizing that there were two distinct objects which produced the echoes. If the two objects are closer than 1.5 mm, the returning echo pulses will merge together and the electronics will see only one wide echo, thus recognizing only one echo-producing object. In general, higher frequency systems can produce narrower outgoing sound wave pulses and, therefore, better axial resolution. Thus a 5-MHz transducer might have an axial resolution of 1.0 mm. This is not a very significant improvement and cannot be expected to make an important difference in the quality of an image. Axial, or depth, resolution does not depend on transducer size or focusing.

Lateral resolution is determined by the width of the beam, which varies with the depth into the patient (Fig. 1-4). If two objects are at the same depth and are closer together than the beam width, they do not produce distinguishable echoes. For two separate objects to produce distinguishable echoes, they must be farther apart than the beam is wide, so that the beam cannot hit them both at once. Thus, lateral resolution is equal to the beam width and is considerably worse than axial resolution. For example, an unfocused 3.5-MHz–1-cm-diameter transducer has an average lateral resolution (beam width) of roughly 8.5 mm between scanning depths of 0 to 15 cm. Compare this with a depth resolution of 1.5 mm.

Sound beams can be focused to make them narrower, thus improving the lateral resolution. Focusing can be accomplished within the electronic circuitry of a phased array system or can be accomplished with a sonic lens, which can be used with any type of transducer. Electronic focusing only works in the plane of the sector scan; therefore, some phased arrays employ a lens to focus in the direction perpendicular to this plane. Some phased array equipment does not utilize electronic focusing at all, but simply uses a sonic lens as the mechanical sector scanners do.

Sound beams cannot be perfectly focused unless the transducer is essentially infinitely large compared to the wavelength of the sound. This condition never exists in medical ultrasound equipment. The best focusing that can be achieved happens such that:

$$\text{focal spot size} \cong \frac{\lambda x}{d}, \tag{1}$$

where x is the distance from the lens-covered transducer to the focal point, λ is the wavelength of the sound wave, and d is the diameter of the transducer. No ultrasound beam can ever be smaller than $\lambda x/d$. This quantity is plotted as a straight line in Figure 1-4 along with the unfocused and lens-focused beam widths of a typical 3.5-MHz transducer (1-cm diameter).

Examination of Figure 1-4 shows some interesting facts. The lens-focused transducer has a beam width which is: (1) within 1 mm of the minimum possible beam width over a range of 6 to 15 cm, (2) within 2 mm of the minimum possible beam width up to 20 cm, and (3) much greater than the minimum possible beam width inside 6 cm. In other words, the lateral resolution obtained is quite good compared to what is theoretically possible, except in the near field.

In pediatric echocardiography there is great interest in the first 5 to 6 cm of scanning depth where the lateral resolution of a typical sector scanner is poor (as shown in Fig. 1-4). There are two ways to gain improved resolution in the near-field region. One way is to use a dynamically focused phased array beam. The other way is to use a higher frequency (i.e., 5 MHz) and smaller transducer (either phased array or mechanical sector scanner).

As noted above, phased arrays are capable of being focused electronically

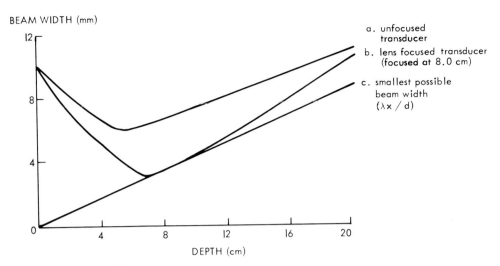

FIG. 1-4. *Beam width: 1.0-cm transducer: 3.5 MHz.* **A.** *Unfocused transducer,* **B.** *lens focused transducer (focused at 8.0 cm), and* **C.** *smallest possible beam width (λx/d).*

in the scan plane (Fig. 1-3b). The transmitted pulse can only be focused at one depth, but the returning pulses can be focused at a number of successive depths. This is a special type of electronic focusing called dynamic focusing. The focal properties of the phased array depend on the phasing of the individual elements. In dynamic focusing, the phasing is changed several times while the electronics is waiting for returning echoes. As an example: (1) when an outgoing pulse is transmitted into the patient, echoes from depths less than 6 cm will return during the first 78 microseconds after the pulse (during this time the transducer phasing is set to focus at 3 cm); (2) echoes from 6 to 14 cm depth will return during the next 104 microseconds (during this time period, the electronic focusing is set for 8 cm); (3) echoes from 14 to 20 cm depth will arrive during the next 78 microseconds, during which time the system focuses at 16 cm depth. That is, the electronics dynamically changes the electronic focus while waiting for returning echoes. Referring to Figure 1-4, we see that focusing (curve b) can give lateral resolution (beam width) quite close to the best obtainable (curve c) in the region of the focal point. Dynamic focusing, therefore, can approximate perfect focusing at all depths. It only works in the sector scan plane but can help a lot. Its effects can be difficult to see in the mid field, somewhat noticeable in the far field, and a substantial improvement in the near field.

Increasing the frequency and reducing transducer size can also give enormously improved resolution in the near field. This is true for all sector scanners, whether phased array or mechanical. Let us first examine the effect of higher frequency alone (i.e., without reducing transducer size).

Equation (1) states that the focal spot size is λx/d. Wavelength and frequency are inversely proportional so that higher frequency means shorter wavelength. Thus, a higher frequency beam can be focused better (i.e., into a narrower beam). Another important relationship is that the angle of beam divergence in the far field, θ, is given by:

$$\sin \theta = 1.22 \left(\frac{\lambda}{d}\right) \tag{2}$$

Thus, higher frequency (i.e., smaller wavelength) means that the beam does not diverge as much. Figure 1-5 shows the different beam widths from 1-cm transducers of 3.5 and 5 MHz, each focused at 8 cm depth. Curve b of Figure 1-5 (3.5 MHz) is identical to curve b of Figure 1-4. Curve a (5 MHz) is definitely better than curve b but is still quite poor in the near field compared to the smallest possible beam width at 5 MHz.

Now let us consider a smaller 5-MHz transducer, with a diameter of 7 mm. Referring to equations (1) and (2), we see that decreasing d means we cannot focus the beam as well and it will diverge more. The dashed curve on Figure 1-6 represents the beam width of our 7-mm–5-MHz transducer. The beam patterns of 1-cm transducers of 3.5 and 5 MHz are shown again for comparison.

Examination of Figure 1-5 shows that we have substantially improved the near-field resolution by both increasing frequency and reducing transducer size. However, the resolution deeper than 5 cm is not as good as it was with a larger 5-MHz transducer.

From the preceding discussion, it should be clear that a dynamically focused phased array with a large 5-MHz transducer would be the pediatric

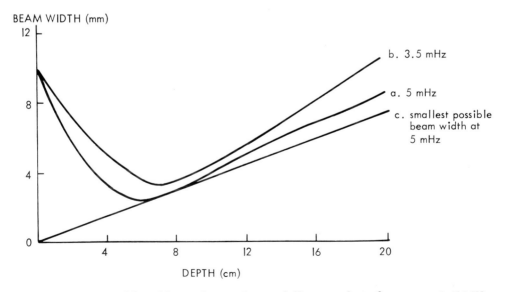

FIG. 1-5. *Beam widths of focused transducers differing only in frequency.* **A.** *5 MHz,* **B.** *3.5 MHz, and* **C.** *smallest possible beam width at 5 MHz.*

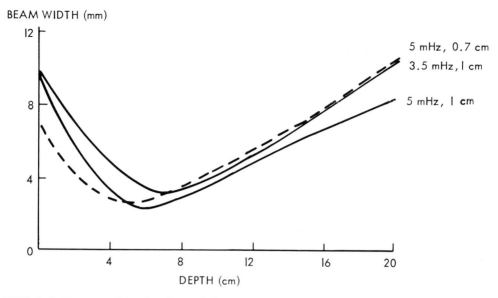

BEAM WIDTH (mm)

5 mHz, 0.7 cm
3.5 mHz, I cm
5 mHz, I cm

DEPTH (cm)

FIG. 1-6. *Beam widths for three different transducers.*

echocardiographer's dream machine from the standpoint of lateral resolution. Unfortunately, there are significant technical problems in creating such a machine. At this time, there is no commercially available phased array of any kind with a transducer frequency higher than 3.5 MHz.

SENSITIVITY

The sensitivity of an ultrasound scanner refers to the system's ability (1) to produce small echoes and (2) to detect small echoes. The ability to detect small echoes depends on the design of the electronics. We will assume, for the purpose of further discussion, that all available scanners have equally good detection sensitivity (which is not necessarily the case) and concentrate on what produces small echoes.

When an ultrasound beam strikes a boundary, an echo is produced. Sound waves, like light waves, obey Snell's Law. The reflected wave (echo) bounces off the boundary at a reflected angle (θ_r) equal to the angle of incidence (θ_i) and in the opposite direction (Fig. 1-7). In other words, unless the sound wave hits the boundary at normal incidence (i.e., perpendicular to the boundary), the echo will not bounce back in the same direction and, therefore, will not return to the transducer for detection.

In cardiac scanning, there are a number of boundaries that can produce echoes. In order of decreasing echo strength, they are:

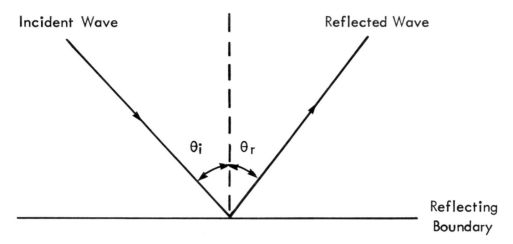

Incident Wave   Reflected Wave

θ_i θ_r

Reflecting
Boundary

FIG. 1-7. *Reflection of ultrasound waves.*

1. Smooth, extensive boundaries where the extent of the boundary is large compared to the wavelength of the sound pulse. Such boundaries are often called specular reflectors and produce strong echoes, but only at normal incidence.

2. Irregular boundaries with ripples where the ripples are somewhat larger than the sound wavelength. An example would be the endocardium, which is characterized by trabeculae. In this case, there will be echoes from the trabeculae even when the sound beam hits the endocardium at large angles of incidence. This is because the sound will almost always find some portion of the trabeculae where it will strike with normal incidence (see Fig. 1-8). Such echoes, however, will be fewer and weaker than those from the specular reflecting boundary described above.

3. Intracellular boundaries where the reflecting surfaces are comparable to, or smaller than, the sound wavelength. Here, one gets quite small reflections, which can, however, be detected by a sensitive instrument. An example of such behavior is the faint but discernible speckled appearance of the interior of the myocardium. It is particularly evident in the interventricular septum in idiopathic hypertrophic subaortic stenosis, where the myocardium has an unusually pronounced crystalline structure.

It is a general principal of physics that scattering (i.e., reflection) of a wave from an object depends on the relative size of the object and the wavelength of the incident wave. When the object is much larger than the wavelength, considerable scattering of the wave occurs. When it is smaller, very little scattering occurs. A simple example involves long ocean swells. As these waves roll past a small object, such as a piling one foot in diameter, they are virtually undisturbed. That is, they hardly see the piling. By contrast, a rock of

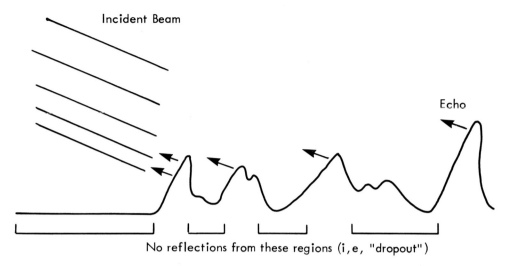

FIG. 1-8. *Reflection from an irregular boundary.*

100 foot diameter will disturb the waves in a very obvious way. This same principle applies to ultrasonic waves. More detectable echoes will come from irregular boundaries or intracellular boundaries with short wavelengths than with longer wavelengths. Shorter wavelengths mean higher frequency. Thus, the ability to produce small echoes (i.e., the sensitivity of an ultrasound system) increases as the transducer frequency is increased.

PENETRATION

The preceding discussions on resolution and sensitivity have a clear message —higher frequency is better. Why then are not all systems high frequency? The answer is attenuation. As sound waves travel into the body, they are attenuated, i.e., they become weaker and weaker as the energy in the beam is dissipated. Unfortunately, attenuation depends on the frequency, and attenuation increases very strongly as the frequency increases. For example, the 10-MHz frequency used in peripheral vascular and ophthalmic ultrasound scanners only penetrates about 3 cm into the body.

There are no simple rules concerning the penetrating power of a sector scanner as a function of frequency. A great deal depends on the sensitivity of the electronics and the transmitted power in the ultrasound beam, which vary from system to system. With more power and higher electronic sensitivity, a system can see deeper into the body at a given frequency. At the present time, most 3.5-MHz systems have enough penetrating power for general pediatric applications and 5-MHz systems enough penetrating power for newborns.

DIGITAL DATA PROCESSING

Digital data processing is relatively new to sector scanning because image data was not stored in digital memory until the last several years. The electronics used to store and display image data in digital form is usually called a digital scan converter. In such a system the data for each individual scan (there are usually 30 such scans per second) fills a digital memory and is displayed. In each successive scan, the old image (i.e., from the previous scan) is dropped from the memory and replaced by the new image. A major advantage of such a system is its ability to freeze the image at any moment. Upon a command from the operator (pushing a button) or from the electronics (i.e., triggering with an ECG trace), the memory simply holds and displays the most recent scan. Even though the sector scanner continues to scan 30 times per second, the digital scan converter refuses to accept new image data to replace the frozen frame until the operator instructs the system to resume real-time scanning. Such freeze frames are considerably superior to the older analog freeze frames, in which the real-time data is recorded on video tape and the image is frozen by stopping the video tape recorder.

The superior freeze frame is sufficient justification for incorporating a digital scan converter into a sector scanner. However, there are other significant advantages. An image stored in a digital scan converter can be manipulated by digital data processing techniques capable of bringing out features in the data that improve its usefulness. Such techniques have long been used in improving nuclear medicine data, satellite images of the earth's surface, telemetry images of moons and planets from deep-space-probing spacecraft, etc. Use of these techniques in ultrasound is in its infancy, and we will only discuss two of the many possible techniques.

As noted earlier in this chapter, the sector scanner's image presentation gets sparser in the far field, where the scan lines become increasingly separated. A digital scan converter can fill in the gaps by interpolation, which means creating artificial scan lines with data that is an average of the data from the nearby actual scan lines. This smooths out the far-field image, making it more easily interpreted by the eye. Interpolation is a form of spatial averaging and is not a cosmetic trick. It can actually result in an image which is closer to what is truly present in the body than a noninterpolated image.

Another potential capability of a digital scan converter is temporal averaging. Often, users of real-time ultrasound scanners are disappointed by the quality of freeze-frame images compared to the live images because the eye-brain combination does some temporal averaging of the successive frames, which results in a more continuous and pleasing image.

Temporal averaging can also help improve image quality. If each successive scan frame were exactly the same, temporal averaging would not be helpful. But each successive frame is not the same. Even in the one-thirtieth second between successive scans, the heart moves slightly. Furthermore, the entire body moves with respiration. Each successive scan sees the heart in a slightly different orientation, and the echo pattern from an irregular surface changes from scan to scan. Even though the changes are not very great, when two successive scans are added together, a smoother, more pleasing (and correct) image is obtained.

The eye and brain always retain a little of recent scan frames, even while seeing the current one. When a simple freeze frame is activated, the residual image of the recent frames dies away and the eye-brain combination sees only the current scan image. The temporal averaging effect is lost and the image does not seem as good. A digital scan converter can temporally average frames electronically, yielding a freeze frame that looks to the eye more comparable to the live image. For example, the scan converter might present the current scan at full intensity, the previous one at one-half intensity, the next earlier one at one-quarter intensity, and so forth. The eye brain combination no longer has to smooth out the image through temporal averaging; the digital scan converter does it instead.

TRANSDUCER SIZE

The size of a transducer and its housing (i.e., a probe) can be important in the practical application of a sector scanner. While the inherent, image-producing capability of a scanner does not depend on probe size (except as discussed with respect to resolution above), probe size can be of great practical consequences. Probe size is very intimately related to the machine–patient and physician–patient interaction. Because cardiac scanning must be done through ultrasonic windows (i.e., the intercostal spaces), a smaller probe will make it possible to obtain a larger number of views in a larger number of patients. Mechanical sector scanners tend to have larger and more unwieldy probes than phased arrays, although design advances are making them smaller.

SIMULTANEOUS M-MODE

The phased array system can perform one or two M-mode studies at the same time as it is producing a two-dimensional image. The phased array can choose the exact direction of an individual scan line electronically; it need not scan lines in sequence from one side of the sector to the other, but can jump around from line to line at will. The user may select the scan line (or lines) along which the M-mode is being obtained and watch the position on the two-dimensional image at the same time. This very convenient feature allows the user to direct the M-mode beam by making use of the image rather than having to watch the M-mode itself.

Present day mechanical sector scanners cannot do simultaneous M-mode because the sector scan lines are swept continuously from one side of the sector scanner to the other. That is, the mechanical systems cannot jump around from line to line at will. There are mechanical sector scanners under design at present that will be capable of doing simultaneous M-modes. They will make use of an extra transducer for this purpose. One transducer will do the M-mode, while another separate system does the two-dimensional image. Then the system can time share between the image and the M-mode, giving the M-mode a sufficient number of pulses per second, just like the phased array scanners now do. Such mechanical sector scanners are not commercially available at this time.

REFERENCE

1. Wells PNT: Biomedical Ultrasonics. London, Academic Press, 1977

CHAPTER 2

Techniques for Performing the Echocardiographic Examination

The acquisition of a good quality, two-dimensional echocardiographic examination requires a thorough knowledge of cardiac anatomy and spatial relations. In infants and children, the acquisition of a successful echocardiographic examination also depends upon the environmental surroundings and the manner in which the child is approached. Some of the techniques that we have found especially useful in examining infants and children are discussed below.

THE ROOM

A quiet and nonthreatening environment is best when examining pediatric patients. The room should have facilities to be darkened (i.e., window shades) and a rheostatic control of the lighting system. In this way, the room can be made light enough to perform the echocardiographic examination and dark enough to display clearly the television monitor. The room should also be warm and well ventilated but not drafty.

Pictures that are of interest to small children should be placed in strategic locations throughout the laboratory to provide a comforting environment as well as a visual distraction to the child while he or she is lying in a particular position. Also, we have found that a decorative mobile hung above the child's head provides a useful distraction during suprasternal notch echocardiography (Fig. 2-1). Music boxes or other forms of music provide an auditory distraction that is sometimes very helpful.

THE BED OR CRIB

The ideal bed is one in which the head of the bed can be raised or lowered and there is access to the child from both sides. Loose pillows can be used to position the patient in the angles required for the various echocardiographic views. On the bed, we use a 20-cm foam rubber mattress with a semicircular hole cut out of the left side (Fig. 2-1). With the patient lying in a left lateral decubitus position over the hole, the transducer can be placed in the hole and applied to the cardiac apex. This technique facilitates apical echocardiography, especially in those patients whose apical impulse is displaced laterally and posteriorly.

For small infants, we use a rubber mattress warmer (the Hamilton Aquamatic) with a rheostatic temperature control (Fig. 2-1). The warmer is placed under the sheet and provides an effective heat source for infants undergoing echocardiographic examination.

In the nursery we prefer to examine small infants in a radiant warmer rather than an isolette because of the greater freedom and access to the patient provided by the former. The isolette makes it difficult to perform complete studies and should be avoided as a place to examine infants if at all possible.

ELECTRODES

We apply electrodes to the infant's back in the regions of the right and left shoulders and the left kidney. With this method, the examiner has access to the entire precordium without being cluttered by wires and electrodes. Also, the wires and electrodes are away from the exploring hands of small children. We use an infant bottle warmer to keep the sonic jelly at a warm temperature so as not to shock the infant by the application of cold jelly on the electrodes or the transducer.

PACIFICATION

Cooperation is necessary for a successful echocardiographic examination. Older children require an explanation of the test and an explanation that they will come to no harm during the study. We sometimes provide the child with a lollipop (if the parents or referring physician do not object) or a small toy in order to gain the child's cooperation. For infants, we have pacifiers available should the child arrive in the laboratory without one. The pacifier can be dipped in raspberry syrup as an added pacification. Feeding is still one of the best pacifiers for small infants, and we encourage parents to complete the infant's feeding prior to the study. In instances when this cannot be done, we keep a supply of sterile water, dextrose water, and processed milk that can be given to the patient before or during the study. It is also important that infants

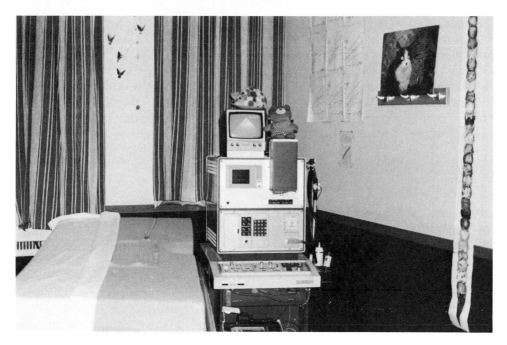

FIG. 2-1. *The pediatric echocardiography laboratory at the University of California at San Francisco.*

not be examined in a soiled diaper as they frequently will not be quiet until they have had their diapers changed.

THE PARENT OR GUARDIAN

We encourage the parent or guardian of the child to be present during the test. This individual can act as the child's companion and source of reassurance, which tends to settle the child and acts as a positive reinforcement for both adult and child. The child is comforted by the parent who in turn is reassured that the child is not coming to harm. The child frequently responds better to the coaxing of a parent to lie in a particular position than he or she would from a technician. The constant supervision of the parent during the study facilitates the cooperation of the child.

SEDATION

Despite all of these ruses, it is sometimes necessary to sedate a fretful child rather than to perform the study under less than optimal circumstances. For sedation, we use chloral hydrate in a dose of 50 to 100 mg/kg depending on how agitated the child is. We do not use more than 1 gm under any circumstance. The child should not be fed milk after administration of chloral hydrate as we have found that this increases the incidence of vomiting. We generally ask the parents to help administer the drug, and, at that time, the parent is informed of the gastrointestinal and central nervous system effects of the drug. We always caution the parent that the child may be disoriented for several hours after the procedure. If the chloral hydrate cannot be given orally, a rectal suppository (300 mg/capsule) is available.

PERSONNEL

It is desirable to keep the number of people in the room at a minimum so as not to arouse the child's concern. In a teaching institution there are always eager students observing studies; if possible, however, these persons should observe the study through a one-way mirror or on a closed-circuit video monitor. Conversation and comments should be kept to a minimum during the procedure as an inadvertent exclamation may lead to considerable anxiety on the part of the child and the parent who are often emotionally charged by the fact that the procedure was indicated.

CHAPTER 3

The Normal Two-Dimensional Echocardiographic Examination

In this chapter, we will describe the structures seen in the standard echocardiographic planes and the techniques used to obtain these planes. The orientation of the views is consistent with the recommendations of the American Society of Echocardiography.[1]

There are two basic planes that can be used to examine the heart and great vessels: (1) a plane parallel to the major axis of the left ventricle and/or the great vessels and (2) a plane perpendicular to the major axis of the left ventricle and/or the great vessels (Figs. 3-1 and 3-2). The echocardiographic planes are slightly offset from the true anatomic planes; hence, they are termed the long axis and short axis planes rather than the sagittal, coronal, or horizontal planes.

To obtain these echocardiographic planes, the transducer can be applied to any of four general areas: (1) the parasternal area in the region of the second, third, or fourth left intercostal spaces, (2) the cardiac apex, (3) the subcostal region, or (4) the suprasternal notch. In each of these areas, the transducer can be applied in a long or short axis plane, and a number of echocardiographic planes can be generated by moving the transducer from side-to-side, top-to-bottom, or clockwise-to-counterclockwise.

In most systems, the video display is oriented with the apex of the sector wedge at the top of the screen and the widest part of the sector wedge at the bottom of the screen. The transducer usually has an index mark that should be oriented either toward the patient's head or the patient's left side. In this manner, as the viewer faces the videoscreen, the patient's cranial structures are always to the right-hand side of the videoscreen, and the patient's right-sided structures are always on the left-hand side of the videoscreen. In this system, the echocardiographic plane is displayed as if the viewer were looking at the cut section of the heart from the patient's left hip.

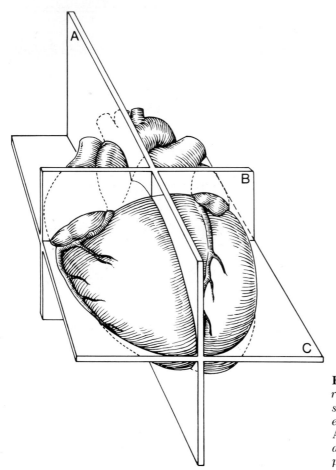

FIG. 3-1. *Diagrammatic representation of the heart showing the approximate echocardiographic planes.* **A.** *long-axis plane;* **B.** *short-axis plane;* **C.** *four-chamber plane.*

In addition to the actual two-dimensional image, it is desirable to display an electrocardiogram for physiologic reference and a scale marker for making measurements. A scale marker is especially important in the echocardiographic examination of the small infant and child where magnification of the image prevents the viewer from being aware of the actual size of the structures. In most of the illustrations in this text, a scale marker is present either on the left-hand side of the photograph or along the right-hand side of the sector wedge (the distance between the dots is 1 cm).

THE PARASTERNAL VIEWS

The parasternal area was the first used for examining the heart.[2,3] These views are generally best obtained with the patient lying in a left lateral decubitus

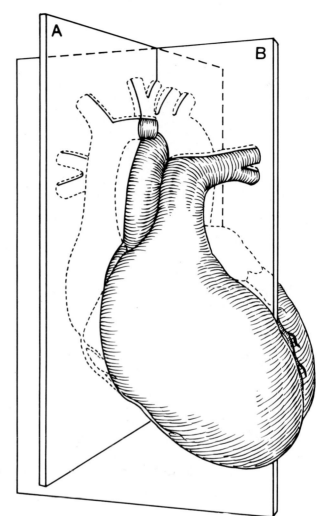

FIG. 3-2. *Diagrammatic representation of the suprasternal planes through the heart.* **A.** *long-axis plane, which defines the ascending aorta, the transverse aorta with the vessels to the head and neck, and the descending aorta.* **B.** *short-axis plane, which defines the innominate veins and superior vena cava, the transverse aorta, the pulmonary arteries, and the left atrium.*

position with slight cranial elevation as for the normal M-mode echocardiographic examination. The transducer is applied close to the sternum in the second, third, or fourth intercostal spaces.

The Parasternal Long-Axis View

The parasternal long-axis view is obtained by orienting the plane along the major axis of the heart from the left hip to the right shoulder (Figs. 3-3 and 3-4). The echoes arising from the transducer bang and the chest wall occupy the apex of the fan. The right ventricular anterior wall is identified below the transducer bang. In the young child, echoes from the thymus may be seen be-

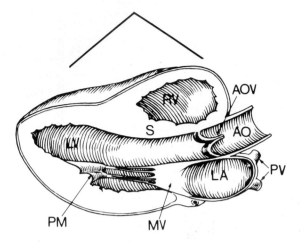

FIG. 3-3. *Diagrammatic repre-sentation of the parasternal long-axis plane. The apex of the heart is displayed to the left and the base of the heart is displayed to the right. The angle above the diagram represents the scanning angle. AO, aorta; AOV, aortic valve; LA, left atrium; LV, left ventricle; MV, mitral valve; PM, papillary muscles; PV, pulmonary veins; RV, right ventricular outflow; S, ventricular septum.*

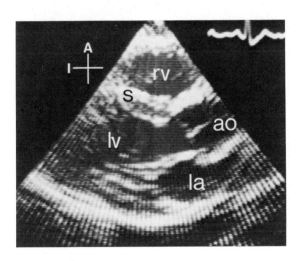

FIG. 3-4. *Parasternal long-axis view in a normal patient. A, anterior; ao, aorta; I, inferior; la, left atrium; lv, left ventricle; rv, right ventricle; S, ventricular septum.*

tween the right ventricular anterior wall and the chest wall. The portion of the right ventricular cavity seen in the standard parasternal long axis plane is the outflow portion of the ventricle. The echoes from the ventricular septum are continuous with the echoes from the anterior aortic root. In this view, the superior portion of the ventricular septum is largely outflow ventricular septum, but a small portion of the membranous septum is seen as well. More of the membranous ventricular septum can be seen by angling the transducer slightly medially.

The outflow and inflow regions of the left ventricle are well defined in the long-axis view. The cardiac apex cannot be seen from the parasternal long-axis view because this view is slightly medial to the apical portion of the ventricle and also because the area subtended by the sector scanner cannot incorporate the entire left ventricle from this location. Posteriorly, the posteromedial papillary muscle can often be seen giving rise to the chordae tendinae, which insert into the anterior and posterior mitral valve leaflets. The anterior mitral valve leaflet is continuous with the posterior aortic root. The origin of the posterior mitral valve leaflet from the area of the atrioventricular groove can be identified. The posterior wall of the left ventricle can be seen behind the papillary muscle and mitral valve leaflets. In the normal heart, a small coronary sinus can often be seen as a circular structure in the region of the atrioventricular groove anterior to the pericardial echo.[4,5] The descending aorta can be seen as an oval to circular structure in the area of the coronary sinus posterior to the pericardial echo.[5] The fact that the descending aorta appears oval or circular rather than longitudinal is an indicator of how far the parasternal long-axis view is from the true sagittal plane.

A portion of the ascending aorta can be seen in the parasternal long-axis view. The aortic valve leaflets can be identified within the aortic root. Usually the region of the corpora arantii can be seen in the center of the aortic root in diastole. The thin bases of the normal valve cusps are more difficult to define. During systole, the leaflets can frequently be seen in the open position close to the walls of the sinuses of Valsalva. The ostium of the right coronary artery can often be seen in the anterior aortic root above the aortic valve.

From the standard parasternal long-axis view, the transducer can be angled slightly medially to image portions of the right ventricular inflow tract or slightly laterally to image portions of the right ventricular outflow tract. When the transducer is angled medially, the aortic root disappears from the image, and the right atrium, right ventricle, and tricuspid valve are seen. A larger portion of the membranous ventricular septum can be imaged by this maneuver. It is even possible to obtain a four-chamber view from the parasternal area (Fig. 3-5). The transducer can also be rotated laterally to image the right ventricular outflow tract, the pulmonary valve, and the main pulmonary artery.

The Parasternal Short-Axis View

From the parasternal long-axis view, the transducer can be rotated 90° clockwise to obtain the parasternal short-axis view. The index mark on the transducer is then to the patient's left side, so that the left-sided structures are seen on the right-hand side of the video screen.[1] The short-axis plane is generally oriented between the right hip and left shoulder. A number of short-axis planes can be obtained depending on the level of the tomographic section (Figs. 3-1 and 3-6). The most caudal angulation of the parasternal short axis plane produces a section through the left ventricular apex,[3] which allows one to evaluate contraction of this segment of the left ventricle. More cranial angulation shows the circular left ventricle. A portion of the right ventricle is seen anteriorly and to the right (Figs. 3-6 and 3-7). The anterolateral and posteromedial papillary muscles can be seen within the left ventricle. The ventricular septum seen at this level consists of portions of the inlet and trabeculated ventricular septum. The portion of the left ventricular wall identified in this

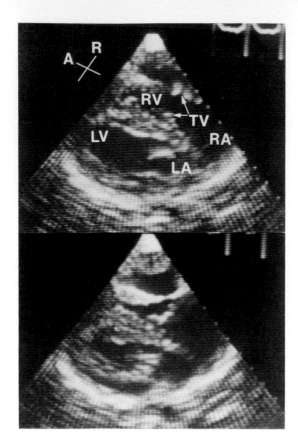

FIG. 3-5. *Parasternal long axis views taken in diastole (**top**) and systole (**bottom**) from a patient with right ventricular (RV) and pulmonary artery hypertension. The transducer was oriented medially and inferiorly from the standard long-axis view in order to image the inflow portion of the right ventricle, the right atrium (RA), and the tricuspid valve (TV). More of the membranous ventricular septum can be seen in this view. A thickened right ventricular anterior wall and prominent anterior papillary muscle of the right ventricle can be seen. A, apex; LA, left atrium; LV, left ventricle; R, right.*

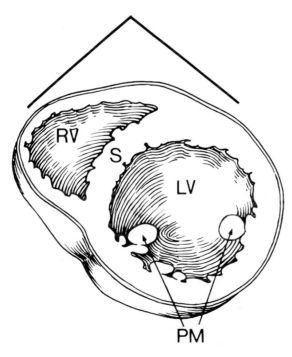

FIG. 3-6. *Diagrammatic representation of a parasternal short-axis plane at the level of the papillary muscles (PM) of the left ventricle (LV). The angle at the top of the figure represents the scanning angle. The left ventricle is circular and contains posteromedial and anterolateral papillary muscles. The ventricular septum (S) separates the left ventricle from the right ventricle (RV).*

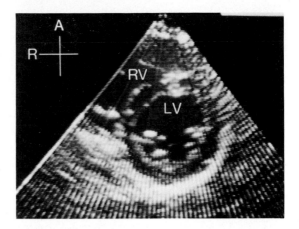

FIG. 3-7. *A parasternal short-axis view through the left ventricle (LV) from a normal patient. A, anterior; R, right; RV, right ventricle.*

plane is a portion of the posterior and lateral wall. In this view, the tricuspid valve can be seen within the right ventricle.

When the image of the left ventricle is circular, the tomographic plane is perpendicular to the major axis of the heart. When the transducer position is too caudal or too cranial, the left ventricular image is elongated. Indeed, a four-chamber view displaying the atria and the ventricles can be obtained from the parasternal area.[2] This parasternal view is a useful intermediate view between the apical four-chamber and subcostal four-chamber views described below.

With slight cranial angulation, the anterior and posterior mitral valve leaflets can be seen in the left ventricle as they open and close during the cardiac cycle. In real time, the alternate opening and closing of the bicommissural valve has the appearance of a fish mouth (Fig. 3-8).

Slightly more cranial angulation displays the left ventricular outflow tract. When enlarged, the coronary sinus can be seen in this plane and should not be mistaken for a posterior pericardial effusion. The circular left ventricular

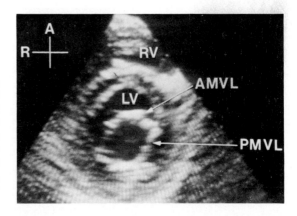

FIG. 3-8. *Parasternal short axis plane at the level of the mitral valve orifice. The left ventricle (LV) appears circular in this plane. The anterior mitral valve leaflet (AMVL) and posterior mitral valve leaflet (PMVL) can be seen within the left ventricle. A, anterior; R, right; RV, right ventricle.*

outflow tract is bordered anteriorly by the ventricular septum and posteriorly by the anterior mitral valve leaflet. The left atrium is seen behind the mitral valve. This portion of the ventricular septum is made up of membranous septum medially and outlet septum laterally. Anterior and to the right, portions of the right ventricle, tricuspid valve, and right atrium can be seen. The interatrial septum can be identified between the two atria.

With more cranial angulation, the right ventricular outflow tract and great vessels can be seen (Fig. 3-9). The short-axis plane at the level of the aortic valve defines several important points of cardiac anatomy (Figs. 3-10 and 3-11). In this view the circular aortic root occupies the center of the fan. In diastole, the three aortic valve cusps form a Y or inverted "Mercedes-Benz" emblem in the aortic root. All three diastolic closure lines may not be seen simultaneously. It is more usual to identify only two of the three diastolic closure lines simultaneously so that a V pattern rather than a Y pattern is seen.

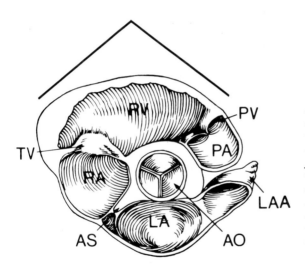

FIG. 3-9. *A diagrammatic representation of the parasternal short-axis view at the level of the aortic valve. The aorta (AO) is seen in cross section with its three cusps forming a Y pattern. The tricuspid valve (TV), pulmonary valve (PV), and atrial septum (AS) are seen. LA, left atrium; LAA, left atrial appendage; PA, pulmonary artery; RA, right atrium; RV, right ventricle.*

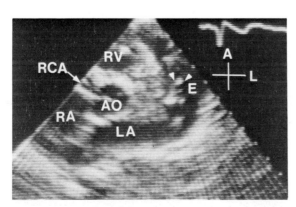

FIG. 3-10. *A parasternal short-axis plane at the level of the aorta (AO) defining the left atrial appendage (arrows). A pericardial effusion (E) highlights the area of the left atrial appendage. The circular aortic root is identified with a prominent right coronary artery (RCA) arising from it. The right ventricular outflow tract is situated anteriorly. The atrial septum divides the left atrium (LA) from the right atrium (RA). A, anterior; L, left; RV, right ventricle.*

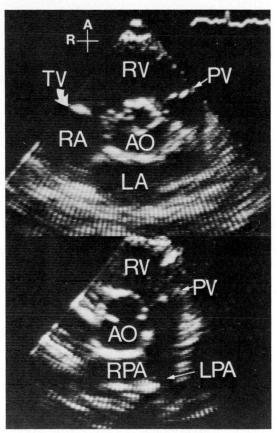

FIG. 3-11. Top. *A parasternal short-axis view through the base of the heart from a normal subject. The aorta (AO) and aortic valve leaflets are seen in cross section in the center of the fan. A portion of the right ventricle (RV) between the tricuspid valve (TV) and the pulmonic valve (PV) is seen anterior to the aorta. A, anterior; LA, left atrium; R, right; RA, right atrium.* **Bottom.** *By angulating the transducer cranially and slightly leftward from the standard parasternal short-axis view, the main pulmonary artery and its bifurcation into right and left pulmonary artery branches (RPA and LPA) can be seen.*

The posterior junction between the left and noncoronary cusps is difficult to image because it is parallel to the plane of sound. The right coronary cusp is seen anteriorly between the septal leaflet of the tricuspid valve and the pulmonary valve. The left coronary cusp lies between the pulmonary valve and the left atrium; and the posterior or noncoronary cusp lies between the left atrium and the tricuspid valve. The interatrial septum is opposite the noncoronary cusp.

The right ventricle appears sausage shaped in this view as it courses anteriorly around the aorta to reach the pulmonary artery. The parts of the right ventricle included in this view are a small portion of the right ventricular inlet and a large portion of the right ventricular outflow area. There are no actual landmarks that can be seen to define these different portions of the right ventricle in the parasternal short-axis view.

To the left and anterior of the aortic valve, the pulmonary valve and a portion of the main pulmonary artery can be seen. Care must be taken not to mistake the adjacent left atrial appendage as part of the main pulmonary artery. Posterior to the aorta, a portion of the left atrium can be visualized.

With medial angulation of the transducer, the septal and anterior tricuspid valve leaflets can be seen. In addition, with medial and inferior angulation of the transducer, larger portions of the right atrium and right ventricle can be identified.

With slight changes in the direction of the plane, it is possible to define more specific features of the pulmonary artery anatomy and coronary artery anatomy. Slight cranial and leftward angulation of the transducer from the standard parasternal short-axis view at the base of the heart displays the pulmonary artery branches more clearly (Fig. 3-11, bottom frame). This view can often be obtained more easily by moving the transducer slightly inferiorly (one intercostal space) and laterally, which brings the right ventricular outflow tract directly beneath the transducer. The pulmonary artery arises and courses almost directly posteriorly. The left pulmonary artery courses in an almost continuous posterior sweep from the main pulmonary artery. The right pulmonary artery, however, arises from the main pulmonary artery and courses to the right behind the aortic root and superior to the upper border of the left atrium. This view of the main pulmonary artery, the pulmonary artery branches, and the ascending aorta provides a useful plane for assessing the absolute pulmonary artery size and the pulmonary artery size relative to the aortic root size.

Although it is possible to image both the right and left coronary arteries simultaneously as they arise from the aortic root, it is often easier to image the coronary arteries separately. In order to image the left coronary artery, the transducer should be angled cranially from the aortic root, and the plane rotated slightly clockwise. This maneuver images the plane in which the coronary artery runs on the surface of the ventricle between the pulmonary artery and the left atrial appendage.[6] Also, portions of the left main coronary artery can be seen while imaging either the pulmonary artery or the left atrial appendage. Ideally, the left coronary artery should be seen from its origin at the aortic root to its bifurcation into the proximal left anterior descending and circumflex arteries (Fig. 3-12). Because the circumflex artery courses anteriorly,

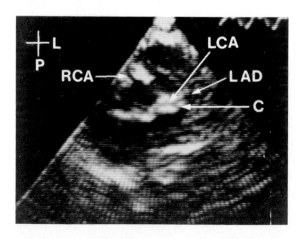

FIG. 3-12. A parasternal short-axis view in a normal patient demonstrating the coronary artery anatomy. This still-frame image was obtained slightly cranial to the aortic valve leaflets and demonstrates the right coronary artery (RCA), the left coronary artery (LCA), and the bifurcation of the LCA into the left anterior descending (LAD) and the circumflex (C) branches. L, left; P, posterior.

it is more difficult to image. In order to visualize the right coronary artery from the short axis view, the transducer should be rotated slightly clockwise and angled slightly cranially from the plane of the aortic valve, thereby allowing a display of a variable length of the right coronary artery as it courses anteriorly on the surface of the ventricle (Fig. 3-10). Too much transducer angulation or rotation can cause failure to visualize the coronary arteries. The resolution of the coronary arteries in the short-axis plane is axial rather than lateral; therefore, they can be well resolved even in neonates.[7]

THE APICAL VIEWS

Initially, the transducer was moved from the parasternal area toward the cardiac apex for examining the left ventricular apex in patients with coronary artery disease. Subsequently, it was discovered that if the transducer were placed directly over the cardiac apex and directed toward the base of the heart, examination of most of the cardiac chambers would be possible. The current nomenclature for describing the apical views is: the apical four-chamber plane (previously called the hemiaxial equivalent view)[8] and the apical long-axis plane (previously called the right anterior oblique equivalent view). With slight cranial or caudal angulation, a spectrum of similar planes, especially four-chamber planes, can be obtained from the apical area.[2]

To obtain accurate transducer placement over the cardiac apex, the apical impulse should be palpated and the transducer should be applied with the same precision as required for apexcardiography. Palpation of the cardiac apex can be facilitated by tilting the patient onto the side of the cardiac apex, usually the left side. This can be done by placing a pillow behind the patient's back. In older patients, raising the head of the bed slightly is also helpful.

The transducer should be applied to the cardiac apex and directed cranially to obtain the apical planes. The back portion of the transducer, especially bulky mechanical scanners, can touch the bed and prevent appropriate transducer placement. In order to circumvent this problem, we use a 20-cm foam rubber mattress with a hole carved out of the side in the region of the cardiac apex (Fig. 2-1). The large hole allows the transducer to be manipulated freely in all directions.

The Apical Four-Chamber View

To obtain the apical four-chamber view, the transducer is directed perpendicular to the atrial and ventricular septa and through the plane of the mitral and tricuspid valves (Figs. 3-13 and 3-14). The transducer is oriented with the index mark pointing towards the patient's left. In this way, the right-sided structures are on the left-hand side of the television screen and the left-handed structures are on the right-hand side of the television screen.

The apical four-chamber view shows the heart divided into its four chambers by the septa and the two atrioventricular valves. The left ventricle occupies more of the apical image than the right ventricle, except in the newborn

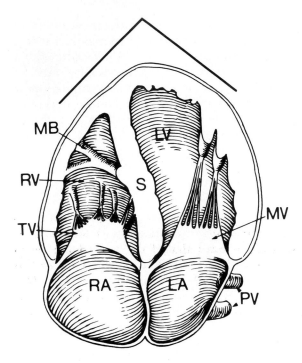

FIG. 3-13. *A diagrammatic representation of the apical four-chamber plane. The angle at the top of the frame represents the scanning angle. The left atrium (LA), left ventricle (LV), right ventricle (RV), and right atrium (RA) are separated by their respective septa and valves. The pulmonary veins (PV) can be seen draining into the left atrium. The moderator band (MB) can be identified within the apex of the right ventricle. MV, mitral valve; S, ventricular septum; TV, tricuspid valve.*

infant where the ventricles occupy an equal share of the cardiac apex. The endocardial outline of the left ventricle is finer than that of the right ventricle because of the differences in the trabeculations of the two ventricles. Coarser trabeculations and the moderator band can usually be seen in the apex of the right ventricle. Occasionally, portions of the papillary muscles can be seen in the right and left ventricle. In the left ventricle, the posteromedial papillary muscle can be identified arising near the septum, and the anterolateral papillary muscle can be seen near the lateral left ventricular wall.

The anterior and septal leaflets of the tricuspid valve and the anterior (medial) and posterior (lateral) leaflets of the mitral valve are seen in the apical four-chamber view. The mitral and tricuspid valves are not situated at exactly the same horizontal level in the apical four-chamber plane. The tricuspid valve is located slightly closer to the cardiac apex than the mitral valve. The supratricuspid portion of the membranous ventricular septum (the atrioventricular portion) is located between the two valves. The lower portion of the ventricular septum seen in this view is the trabeculated septum, and the upper portion of the septum adjacent to the atrioventricular valves is the inlet septum. The left ventricular wall in this view is the lateral left ventricular wall, and the right ventricular wall is the anterior right ventricular wall.

The interatrial septum runs between the atrioventricular valves and the posterosuperior atrial wall. The middle portion of the interatrial septum is frequently not imaged because this region of the septum (the fossa ovalis) is thin

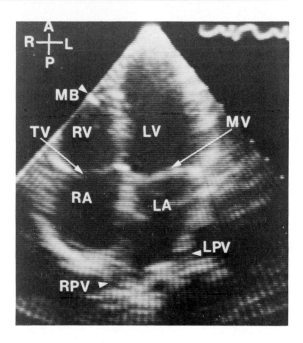

FIG. 3-14. *An apical four-chamber view from a normal patient. The ventricular and atrial septa are seen separating the right- from the left-sided chambers. The tricuspid (TV) and mitral valves (MV) are clearly identified. The tricuspid and mitral valves are not on the same horizontal level; instead, the tricuspid valve is closer to the cardiac apex than the mitral valve. The moderator band (MB) can be seen as a bright echo in the apex of the right ventricle (RV). The pulmonary veins (RPV and LPV) can be seen entering the left atrium (LA). A, anterior; L, left; LV, left ventricle; P, posterior; R, right; RA, right atrium.*

and because the sound beam is parallel to this portion of the atrial septum. In real time, the atrial septum often moves from side to side with phasic differences in interatrial pressure. Such movement may be erroneously interpreted as an atrial septal aneurysm (Fig. 3-15).

A right and a left pulmonary vein can be seen draining into the left atrium (Fig. 3-14). Anterior and lateral to the pulmonary veins, the connection of the left atrial appendage with the body of the left atrium can be identified sometimes, especially with anterior angulation of the transducer. The coronary sinus can be identified along the lateral wall of the left atrium running in the atrioventricular groove.

Except when the eustachian valve can be seen, the right atrium has no particular characteristic features. The eustachian valve is often more prominent in small children. In real time the valve can be seen moving back and forth and should not be mistaken for a foreign body. The site of attachment of the eustachian valve marks the junction of the inferior vena cava with the atrium.

In the apical four-chamber view, the descending aorta can sometimes be identified behind the heart where it appears as a circular structure posterolateral to the left atrium. On occasion, it can be so close to the atrium that it can be falsely interpreted as the coronary sinus or a left atrial membrane. The aorta, however, lies outside the left atrial pericardium.[5,9]

Cranial and caudal tilting of the transducer show different anatomic structures. The coronary sinus can be identified with extreme caudal angulation as it courses from left to right in the atrioventricular groove.[10] Cranial angulation

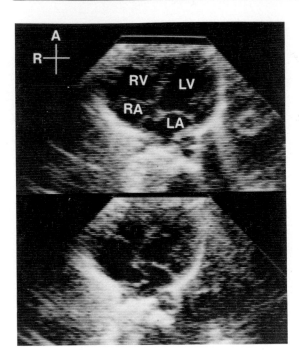

FIG. 3-15. *An apical four-chamber view in a newborn infant demonstrating the motion of the atrial septum. In the upper frame, the atrial septum bulges toward the right atrium (RA). In the lower frame, the atrial septum bulges toward the left atrium (LA). This phasic motion is related to phasic differences in atrial pressure during the cardiac cycle. A, anterior; LV, left ventricle; R, right; RV, right ventricle.*

from the standard apical four-chamber view shows the membranous ventricular septum, the left ventricular outflow tract, and frequently the aortic valve. In addition, with extreme cranial angulation, the right ventricular outflow tract and pulmonary valve can be identified from the apical plane.[8]

The Apical Long-Axis View

The apical long-axis view can be obtained by rotating the transducer 90° counterclockwise from the apical four-chamber view (Figs. 3-1, 3-16, and 3-17). The echocardiographic plane is directed through the major axis of the left ventricle[2,11] and through the planes of the mitral and aortic valves. The portions of the ventricular septum seen in this view are primarily trabeculated and outlet septa. The left ventricular outflow tract, aortic valve, and ascending aorta can also be identified. The left atrium can be seen behind the mitral valve. When examining adult patients some echocardiographers prefer a more caudal long-axis view, which excludes the ascending aorta and aortic root and allows better visualization of the left ventricular anterior wall.

There are marked similarities between the apical and the parasternal long axis planes. However, the apical long-axis view provides a plane more oriented along the major axis of the left ventricle and through the cardiac apex. Also, the left ventricular outflow tract and aortic valve are more perpendicular to the direction of the sound beam in the apical long-axis view, hence,

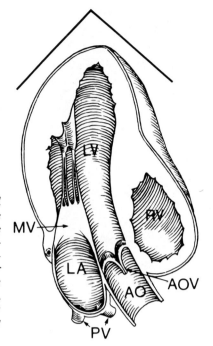

FIG. 3-16. *A diagram representing the apical long-axis plane. The angle at the top of the figure demonstrates the sector scanning angle. This plane passes through the left ventricular apex, defining the cavity of the left ventricle (LV), the posteromedial papillary muscle, the left ventricular wall, and the ventricular septum. The mitral valve (MV), the left atrium (LA), the aortic valve (AOV), the aortic root (AO), and a small portion of the right ventricle (RV) are also seen. PV, pulmonary veins.*

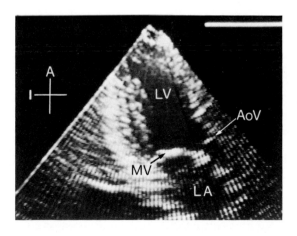

FIG. 3-17. *An apical long-axis view from a normal patient. The apex of the left ventricle (LV) is in the apex of the fan. The posterior wall of the left ventricle and the posteromedial papillary muscle are identified on the left of the figure. The mitral valve (MV) separates the left ventricle from the left atrium (LA). Note that the mitral valve is continuous with the posterior aortic root and the ventricular septum is continuous with the anterior aortic root. The aortic valve (AoV) separates the left ventricle from the ascending aorta. A, apex; I, inferior.*

allowing for more axial resolution of these structures. The superior border of the left atrium is often more clearly visualized in the apical rather than the parasternal long-axis view.

With slight medial rotation from the apical long-axis view, the descending aorta can be seen behind the left ventricle and left atrium (Fig. 3-18).[9]

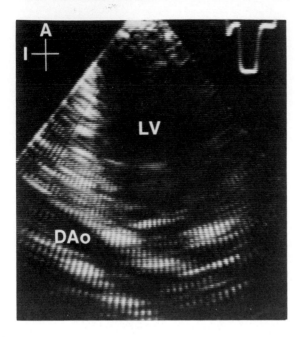

FIG. 3-18. *With slight medial rotation of the transducer from the apical long-axis view, the descending aorta (DAo) can be seen posterior to the left ventricle (LV). A, apex; I, inferior.*

THE SUBCOSTAL VIEWS

The subcostal area allows imaging of a large section of the heart and great vessels.[2,12,13] The structures imaged may be either supra- or infradiaphragmatic.

For the subcostal examination, the patient should be lying in the supine position. A pillow can be placed under the patient's back to increase the degree of lordosis and facilitate the examination from this position. In older patients, the legs can be flexed at the knees and hips to diminish the tension of the abdominal muscles.

It is important while performing the subcostal examination to be cognizant of two factors. First, if one presses the transducer too deeply into the abdomen in small infants, the inferior vena cava can be partially occluded and cause diminished venous return and decreased cardiac output. We have noted a fall in transcutaneous oxygen tension with too vigorous subcostal transducer application in small infants. Second, the abdomen may be tender, and too vigorous a transducer application can cause considerable discomfort. This situation often occurs in postsurgical patients and patients with a distended liver due to cardiac failure. In these situations, subcostal images can be obtained by placing the transducer lower than the free edge of the liver or in an alternative subcostal position.

The Subcostal Views of the Abdomen

For imaging the abdominal aorta and inferior vena cava, the transducer is oriented in the subcostal space in a sagittal body plane. To image the abdominal aorta in its long axis, the transducer is angled toward the left paravertebral gutter. The descending aorta can be seen from above the diaphragm to the bifurcation into the iliac arteries. Usually, only the superior portion of the abdominal aorta is visualized (Fig. 3-19, top). As the position of the descending aorta may vary from patient to patient, a sweep from left to right in the long

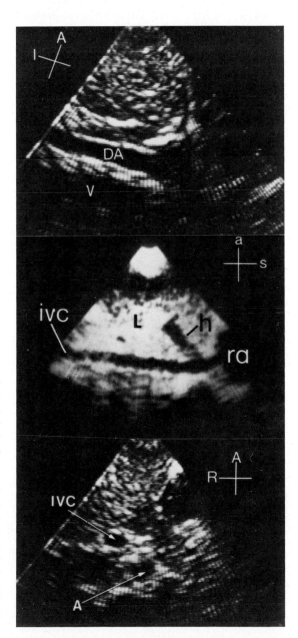

FIG. 3-19. Top. *Subcostal long-axis plane through the descending aorta (DA). The vertebral bodies (V) are seen posterior to the descending aorta. Note the liver echoes anterior to the descending aorta. A, anterior; I, inferior.* **Middle.** *A subcostal long axis view through the inferior vena cava (ivc) and hepatic vein (h). Note the junction of the inferior vena cava with the right atrium (ra). a, anterior; L, liver; s, superior.* **Bottom.** *The horizontal section through the descending aorta (A) and inferior vena cava (IVC) in the abdomen. Note the position of the descending aorta to the left and posterior to the inferior vena cava. A, anterior; R, right.*

axis is necessary to identify the aorta. It is frequently helpful (especially in younger children) to identify the vertebral bodies as the aorta is closely related to them.

From the subcostal view of the descending aorta, the transducer can be angled toward the patient's right to visualize the inferior vena cava (Fig. 3-19, middle). To image the inferior vena caval-right atrial junction, slight cranial angulation and clockwise rotation of the transducer is usually necessary because of the oblique course of the upper portion of the inferior vena cava.

The inferior vena cava, descending aorta, and vertebral bodies can be seen in cross section by placing the transducer in the subcostal space in a horizontal body plane (Fig. 3-19, bottom). Normally, the inferior vena cava is to the right and anterior of the descending aorta. The descending aorta is normally located to the left of the vertebral body and posterior to the inferior vena cava.

The Subcostal Views of the Heart

For imaging the heart from the subcostal plane, there are two basic planes, the short axis and the four-chamber planes. In actuality both of these are a compound of a number of planes, as with the parasternal and apical planes.

The Subcostal Short-Axis View

The subcostal short-axis view is obtained by angling the transducer cranially from the long axis view of the inferior vena cava (Figs. 3-20 and 3-21). In this view, the inferior vena cava can be seen entering the right atrium and bordered by the eustachian valve. This structure has variable length and is more

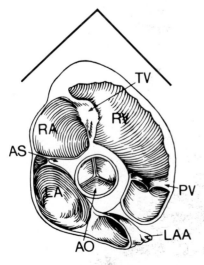

FIG. 3-20. *Diagram of a subcostal short-axis plane through the base of the heart. The angle at the top of the picture is the scanning angle. Note the centrally located aorta (AO) with its valve leaflets. The pulmonary valve (PV), tricuspid valve (TV), and atrial septum (AS) can be seen. The right atrium (RA), right ventricle (RV), left atrium (LA), and left atrial appendage (LAA) also can be seen.*

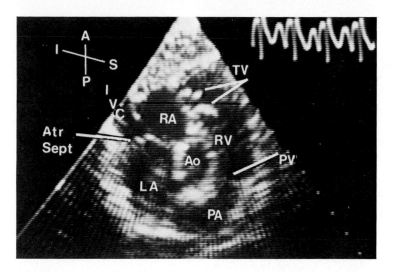

FIG. 3-21. *A subcostal short-axis plane from a normal patient. The inferior vena cava (IVC) is separated from the right atrium (RA) by a prominent eustachian valve. The tricuspid valve (TV) separates the right atrium from the right ventricle (RV), and the pulmonary valve (PV) separates the right ventricle from the pulmonary artery (PA). The central aorta (Ao) is seen. The atrial septum (Atr Sept) divides the right atrium from the left atrium (LA). A, anterior; I, inferior; P, posterior; S, superior.*

prominent in younger children. The atrial septum is perpendicular to the plane of sound and is well imaged. The diaphragmatic surfaces of the right atrium and right ventricle are separated from the transducer by the liver and the diaphragm. By angling the transducer slightly cranially and toward the left, a large part of the body of the right ventricle and the right ventricular outflow tract can be seen. Also, the pulmonary valve, main pulmonary artery, and pulmonary artery branches can be imaged.

The circular aortic root and valve are seen in the center of the fan. The tricuspid valve, pulmonic valve, and atrial septum radiate from the central aorta like the spokes of a wheel. The left atrium in this view is bordered by the atrial septum anteriorly, the aortic root and pulmonary artery laterally, and the free left atrial wall posteriorly and medially.

The superior vena cava–right atrial junction can be seen by angling the transducer slightly cranially, rightward, and superiorly. The left ventricle can be imaged by rotating the transducer leftward and inferiorly from the standard subcostal short axis view. This view (Fig. 3-22) is similar to the parasternal short axis view of the left ventricle. The differences between these views are the angle from which they are obtained and the closeness of the heart to the transducer. Also, the subcostal short-axis view of the left ventricle shows more of the right ventricle and has the ventricular septum parallel to the plane of sound.

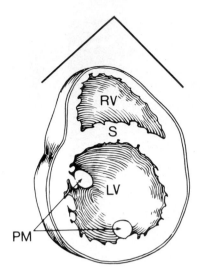

FIG. 3-22. *A diagrammatic representation of the subcostal short axis plane through the left ventricle. The angle at the top of the figure represents the apex of the fan. LV, left ventricle; PM, papillary muscles; RV, rght ventricle; S, septum.*

The Subcostal Four-Chamber View

To obtain the subcostal four-chamber view, the transducer is rotated 90° clockwise from the subcostal short-axis view. From this plane (plane C of Fig. 3-1), the transducer can be angled posteriorly and anteriorly.

In the most posterior plane, all four chambers of the heart can be seen (Figs. 3-23 and 3-24). The subcostal four-chamber view provides essentially

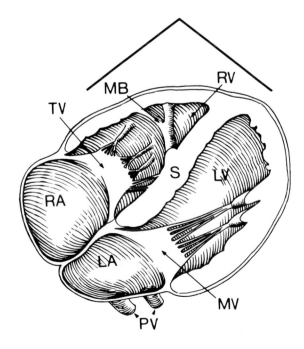

FIG. 3-23. *A diagram of the subcostal four-chamber plane. The angle at the top of the picture represents the scanning angle. LA, left atrium; LV, left ventricle; MB, moderator band; MV, mitral valve; PV, pulmonary veins; RA, right atrium; RV, right ventricle; S, septum; TV, tricuspid valve.*

FIG. 3-24. *A subcostal four-chamber plane from a normal patient. The liver echoes are identified anterior to the right ventricle (RV). The tricuspid (TV) and mitral valve (MV) echoes can be identified. The atrial septum can be seen separating the right atrium (RA) from the left atrium (LA). The pulmonary veins (PV) can be seen entering the left atrium in this plane. A, anterior; I, inferior; LV, left ventricle; P, posterior; S, superior.*

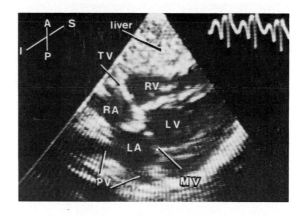

the same structural information as the apical four-chamber view; however, there are important differences in the two views. In the subcostal view, the cardiac apex points to the side; therefore, this view is helpful for defining the position of the cardiac apex (see Chapter 14). The cardiac septa are incident to the plane of sound in the subcostal four-chamber view; therefore, the resolution of these structures is better in this plane. The disadvantages of the subcostal four-chamber view are that it does not image as much of the right ventricle as does the apical four-chamber view and that the alignment of the atrioventricular valves is not as easily defined. Especially in older patients,[10] the subcostal view can be more difficult to obtain than the apical four-chamber view.

The transducer can be angled anteriorly from the four-chamber view to obtain a plane through the left ventricular outflow tract. Portions of the ascending aorta, aortic arch, and descending aorta can be identified.[12] Even more cranial angulation defines the right ventricular outflow tract and the pulmonary arteries (Figs. 3-25 A and B). The crista supraventricularis and the supracristal portion of the right ventricle can be imaged in this view (Fig. 3-25B).

THE SUPRASTERNAL NOTCH VIEWS

The suprasternal notch provides a valuable area for examination of the aortic arch, the pulmonary arteries, and the systemic veins.[2,14-18] For the suprasternal examination, the patient lies supine with a pillow placed beneath the shoulders so as to extend the neck without producing tension on the sternocleidomastoid muscles. In infants and smaller children, it is often helpful to have an assistant place his or her hand firmly beneath the scapulae and lift the back forward slowly and gently so as not to alarm the child. The head may have to be turned slightly toward one side in order to allow appropriate transducer application.

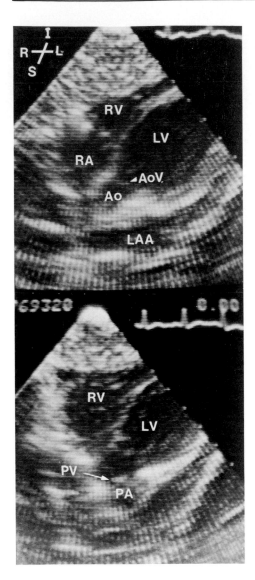

FIG. 3-25. Top. *Subcostal view obtained with cranial angulation of the transducer from the standard subcostal four-chamber plane. The aortic valve (AoV) can be seen separating the aorta (Ao) from the left ventricle (LV). The right atrium (RA) and right ventricle (RV) lie anteriorly next to the liver. The left atrial appendage (LAA) is seen adjacent to the aortic root. I, inferior; L, left; R, right; S, superior.* **Bottom.** *More cranial angulation from the subcostal four-chamber plane shows a large portion of the right ventricle. The pulmonary valve (PV) and pulmonary artery (PA) can be seen continuous with the right ventricle (RV). The area of the crista supraventricularis separates the right ventriclar outflow tract from the body of the right ventricle. The left ventricle (LV) can be identified posterior to the right ventricle in this plane.*

In smaller infants it may not be necessary to place the entire transducer in the suprasternal notch. An adequate view of the aortic arch can be achieved by placing the transducer directly over the manubrium sternum which, because it is cartilaginous, allows transmission of the sound.

In order to keep the younger patient's head extended appropriately, pictures or objects of interest can be placed at strategic points to maintain the child's attention elsewhere during the examination. There are two basic planes that can be obtained for suprasternal notch examination (Fig. 3-2).

Suprasternal Long-Axis View

To obtain the suprasternal long-axis view, the transducer is positioned in the suprasternal notch with the plane oriented between the right nipple and left scapular tip.[17] The index mark is pointing cranially and toward the bed. In this plane the ascending aorta, aortic arch, the vessels to the head and neck, and the descending aorta are seen in longitudinal section. The right pulmonary artery and the right mainstem bronchus are seen in cross section beneath the aortic arch (Figs. 3-26, 3-27, and 3-28). The right bronchus is a circular area that is air filled and, therefore, densely echo reflective. Because it is an eparterial structure, the right bronchus is always imaged in this plane above the right pulmonary artery. Anteriorly, the innominate vein can be seen in cross

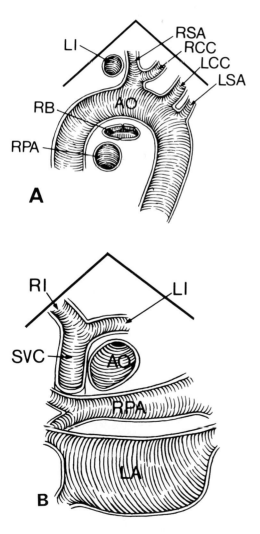

FIG. 3-26. A. *A diagrammatic representation of the suprasternal long-axis plane through the aorta (AO). The angle at the top of the image represents the scanning angle. The ascending aorta, transverse aorta, and descending aorta are seen in longitudinal section. The right pulmonary artery (RPA) and right main stem bronchus (RB) are seen in cross section beneath the aortic arch. The left innominate vein (LI) is seen above the aorta in cross section. The right subclavian (RSA), right common carotid (RCC), left common carotid (LCC), and left subclavian arteries (LSA) are identified arising from the aortic arch.* **B.** *A suprasternal short-axis plane obtained at approximately 90° to the suprasternal long-axis plane. The angle at the top of the figure represents the scanning angle. The right innominate and left innominate veins (RI and LI) are seen joining to form the superior vena cava (SVC). The transverse aorta (AO) is seen in cross section. Posteriorly, the right pulmonary artery (RPA) is seen from its origin from the main pulmonary artery on the right-hand side of the figure to its branches in the hilum of the right lung. Posterior to this, the left atrium (LA) can be identified.*

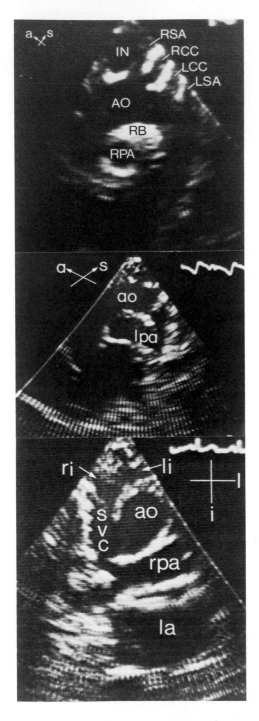

FIG. 3-27. Top. *Suprasternal long-axis view from a normal patient. The right subclavian (RSA), right common carotid (RCC), left common carotid (LCC), and left subclavian arteries (LSA) can be seen arising from the transverse aorta (AO). The right pulmonary artery (RPA) and right bronchus (RB) are seen in cross section beneath the aortic arch. The left innominate vein (IN) can be seen anterior to the transverse aorta. a, anterior; s, superior.* Middle. *A suprasternal long-axis view from a normal patient obtained by tilting the transducer slightly leftward in order to image the left pulmonary artery (lpa). The main and left pulmonary arteries are seen in tangential section as a comma-shaped structure alongside the transverse and descending aorta (ao). a, anterior; s, superior.* Bottom. *A suprasternal short axis plane from a normal patient. The left innominate (li) and right innominate (ri) veins are seen joining to form the superior vena cava (SVC). The transverse aorta (ao) can be seen in cross section. Beneath the transverse aorta, the right pulmonary artery (rpa) can be seen from its origin in the main pulmonary artery on the right-hand side of the image to its branches on the left-hand side of the image. Posterior to the right pulmonary artery, the left atrium (la) can be seen. i, inferior; l, left.*

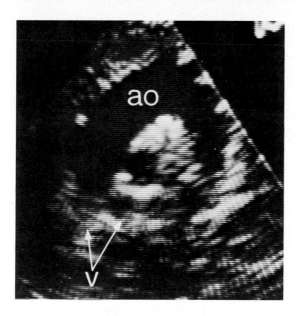

FIG. 3-28. *Suprasternal long-axis plane showing the entire aortic arch (ao) and the aortic valve (v).*

section as it courses from left to right to join in forming the superior vena cava. The left atrium lies posterior to the pulmonary artery.

By tilting the transducer toward the patient's left in the long-axis plane, the left pulmonary artery, transverse aorta, and descending aorta can be seen (Fig. 3-27). In this view, the main pulmonary artery bulb and the left pulmonary artery are imaged tangentially as a comma-shaped structure. The circular part of the comma is the main pulmonary artery and the tail of the comma is the left pulmonary artery branch. Since the left main stem bronchus is hyparterial, there is no bronchial tissue between the left pulmonary artery and the transverse aorta. The relationships between the left and right pulmonary arteries and bronchi assume importance in the differentiation of situs (see Chapter 14).

The Suprasternal Short-Axis View

The suprasternal short-axis view is obtained by rotating the transducer clockwise into a coronal body plane. The index mark points to the patient's left side. In the suprasternal short-axis view, the transverse aorta can be seen in cross section as a circular anterior structure (Figs. 3-26B and 3-27, bottom). The right and left innominate veins join to form the superior vena cava on the right side of the transverse aorta. The lower portion of the superior vena cava passes anteriorly out of the plane. The right pulmonary artery is seen in longitudinal section beneath the transverse aorta. The right pulmonary artery can be seen from its origin in the main pulmonary artery to the division into its branches (Fig. 3-27). Inferior to the pulmonary artery, the left atrium can be identified. With slight anterior angulation of the transducer from the standard short-axis view, the superior vena caval-right atrial junction can be imaged. Often, the entire ascending aorta and aortic valve leaflets can be seen alongside the superior vena cava (Fig. 3-29).

THE FETAL ECHOCARDIOGRAM

Recent publications[19-21] have shown that the heart can be imaged in utero from a variety of planes. Surprisingly good resolution of structures can be obtained from about 16 to 18 weeks of gestation to term. Growth curves for cardiac structures during the last part of pregnancy have been obtained.[20,21] The fetal lie makes imaging in orthodox planes difficult since the fetus often has its back toward the transducer. The echocardiographer has to determine the position of the fetus' head, back, and limbs in order to establish the cranial-caudal and left-right directions. During the fetal echocardiogram, we attempt three basic planes of examination: long-axis, short-axis, and the four-chamber views. Images similar to the long-axis, short-axis, and four-chamber views in the newborn can be obtained (Figs. 3-30 and 3-31). In addition, the aortic arch and the descending thoracic aorta can be seen. In the future, it is clear that this tool will become an additional resource of the genetic counsellor. For example, if a fetus were suspected of having a complete atrioventricular canal defect, tricuspid atresia, or aortic atresia, an image such as that produced in Figure 3-30 or 3-31 could exclude these diagnoses with certainty. To date, fetal studies are still in their "embryonic" stages, and we do not yet have sufficient experience in the use of echocardiography as a diagnostic tool in utero.

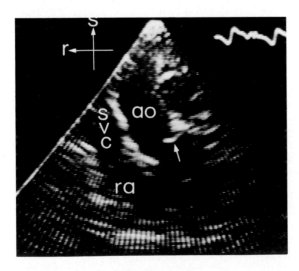

FIG. 3-29. *Suprasternal short axis plane from a normal patient obtained by tilting the transducer anteriorly. This demonstrates the ascending aorta (ao), the aortic valve (arrow), and the left ventricle. The main pulmonary artery is seen to the left of the aorta. To the right, the junction of the superior vena cava (svc) and the right atrium (ra) can be seen. r, right; s, superior.*

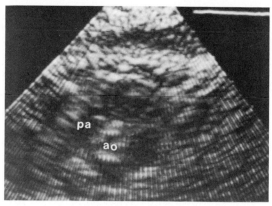

FIG. 3-30. *A parasternal short-axis view from a fetus at 20 weeks gestation. The aorta (ao) and pulmonary artery (pa) are seen in the normal circle-sausage arrangement. In this example, the image is reversed because the index mark was reversed.*

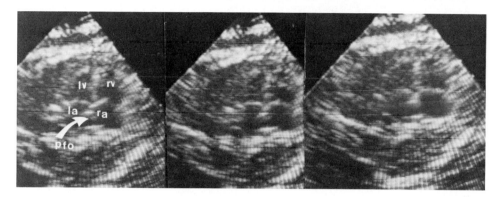

FIG. 3-31. *A series of four-chamber views obtained from a 24-week-old fetus. The four-chamber views are reversed because the fetus was lying upside down and the transducer direction was opposite to normal. In the four-chamber plane, the left atrium (la), left ventricle (lv), patent foramen ovale (Pfo), right atrium (ra), and right ventricle (rv) can be seen. In these three sequences, changes in the sizes of the chambers occur because of cardiac motion.*

REFERENCES

1. Henry WL, DeMaria A, Gramiak R, et al.: Report of the American Society of Echocardiography Committee on Nomenclature and Standards in Two-Dimensional Echocardiography. Circulation 62: 212, 1980
2. Tajik AJ, Seward JB, Hagler DJ, Mair DD: Two-dimensional real-time ultrasonic imaging of the heart and great vessels: Technique, image orientation, structure identification and validation. Mayo Clin Proc 53: 271, 1978
3. Feigenbaum H: Echocardiography. Philadelphia, Lea and Febiger, 1981, p.51

4. Snider AR, Ports TA, Silverman NH: Venous anomalies of the coronary sinus: Detection by M-mode, two-dimensional and contrast echocardiography. Circulation 60: 721, 1979

5. Mintz GS, Kotler MN, Segal BL, Parry WR: Two-dimensional echocardiographic recognition of the descending thoracic aorta. Am J Cardiol 44: 232, 1979

6. Weyman AE, Feigenbaum H, Dillon JC, Johnston KW, Eggelton RC: Non-invasive visualization of the left main coronary artery by cross-sectional echocardiography. Circulation 54: 169, 1976

7. Fisher EA, Sepehri B, Lendrum B, Luken J, Levitsky S: Two-dimensional echocardiographic visualization of the left coronary artery in anomalous origin of the left coronary artery from the pulmonary artery: Pre- and postoperative studies. Circulation 63: 698, 1981

8. Silverman NH, Schiller NB: Apex echocardiography: A two-dimensional technique for evaluation of congenital heart disease. Circulation 57: 503, 1978

9. Seward JB, Tajik AJ: Non-invasive visualization of the entire thoracic aorta: A new application of wide-angle two-dimensional sector echocardiographic technique. Am J Cardiol 43: 387, 1979

10. Bansal RC, Tajik AJ, Seward JB, Offord MS: Feasibility of detailed two-dimensional echocardiographic examination in adults. Mayo Clin Proc 55: 291, 1980

11. Schiller NB, Silverman NH: Two-dimensional ultrasonic cardiac imaging. In Kleid JJ, Arvan SB (eds): Echocardiography: Interpretation and Diagnosis. New York, Appleton, 1978, p.365

12. Bierman FZ, Williams RG: Subxyphoid two-dimensional imaging of the interatrial septum in infants and neonates with congenital heart disease. Circulation 60: 80, 1979

13. Lange LW, Sahn DJ, Allen HD, Goldberg SJ: Subxyphoid cross-sectional echocardiography in infants and children with congenital heart disease. Circulation 59: 513, 1979

14. Goldberg BB: Suprasternal ultrasonography. JAMA 215: 245, 1971

15. Goldberg BB: Ultrasonic measurement of the aortic arch, right pulmonary artery and left atrium. Radiology 101: 383, 1971

16. Allen HD, Goldberg SJ, Sahn DJ, Ovitt TW, Goldberg BB: Suprasternal notch echocardiography: Assessment of its clinical utility in pediatric cardiology. Circulation 55: 605, 1977

17. Sahn DJ, Allen HD, McDonald G, Goldberg SJ: Real-time cross-sectional echocardiographic diagnosis of coarctation of the aorta: A prospective study of echocardiographic-angiographic correlations. Circulation 56: 762, 1977

18. Snider AR, Silverman NH: Suprasternal notch echocardiography: A two-dimensional technique for evaluating congenital heart disease. Circulation 63: 165, 1981

19. Kleinman CS, Hobbins JC, Jaffe CC, Lynch DC, Talner NS: Echocardiographic studies on the human fetus: Prenatal diagnosis of congenital heart disease and cardiac dysrhythmias. Pediatrics 65: 1059, 1980

20. Sahn DJ, Lange LW, Allen HD, et al.: Quantitative real-time cross-sectional echocardiography in the developing normal human fetus and newborn. Circulation 62: 588, 1980

21. Lange LW, Sahn DJ, Allen HD, et al.: Qualitative real-time cross-sectional echocardiographic imaging of the human fetus during the second half of pregnancy. Circulation 62: 799, 1980

CHAPTER 4

Two-Dimensional Contrast Echocardiography

In the late 1960s, Gramiak and Shah[1] first described the echocardiographic contrast effect produced by the injection of indocyanine green dye during cardiac catheterization. With selective injections of this dye, dextrose water, saline, or the patient's own blood, the echocardiographic appearance of various cardiac chambers and structures was confirmed.[2] Subsequent investigators have used contrast echocardiography in cardiac catheterization and by peripheral venous injection to visualize intracardiac flow patterns and to detect shunts.[3-7] The recent application of contrast techniques to the two-dimensional echocardiographic examination has been especially useful for structure validation and for the evaluation of complex congenital cardiac malformations.[8]

It is believed that tiny gas bubbles which are suspended in the contrast liquid act as specular reflectors of ultrasound and give rise to contrast echoes. Various investigators have suggested that these microbubbles form by cavitation at the catheter or needle tip during forceful injections[9] or are caused by the injection of small amounts of gas trapped in the injecting apparatus.[10] Recent studies by Meltzer and colleagues[11] suggest that microbubbles present in the injectant are the source of the contrast effect.

The cloud of echoes produced by the contrast injection follows the downstream flow of blood within the heart. Microbubbles giving rise to the contrast effect are completely filtered by the systemic and pulmonary capillary beds. Thus, contrast echoes will not appear in the left heart following a systemic venous injection unless an intracardiac or intrapulmonary right-to-left shunt is present. Similarly, contrast echoes will not appear in the right heart following a left heart injection unless an intracardiac left-to-right shunt is present.

Peripheral venous contrast echocardiography can be performed using the superficial veins of the scalp, arms, or feet. In our laboratory, a 23- or 25-gauge needle is placed in the vein and connected by a stopcock to two 3-cc syringes filled with bacteriostatic normal saline (Fig. 4-1). We have found that vigorous shaking of the vial of saline prior to filling the syringes enhances the contrast effect, probably by increasing the amount of microbubbles in the solution. For the contrast injection, 0.5 to 3 cc of saline are rapidly injected with a force similar to that of a good hand angiogram from the first syringe followed by a similar injection from the second syringe. Thus, for the newborn infant, a contrast echocardiogram can be obtained with a total of only 1 cc of saline. In larger patients, the contrast effect can be enhanced by squeezing or elevating the extremity after the contrast injection to liberate microbubbles that adhere to the vessel endothelium. In patients old enough to cooperate, the contrast effect can be enhanced by injecting both syringes of saline, while the patient performs a Valsalva maneuver, and observing the echocardiogram during the release phase of the Valsalva maneuver. The following examples were chosen to illustrate the usefulness of two-dimensional contrast echocardiography in the evaluation of infants and children with congenital heart disease.

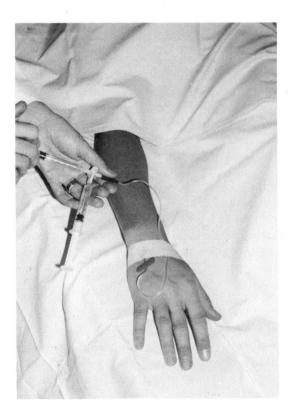

FIG. 4-1. *Method used to perform contrast echocardiography. A 23- or 25-gauge needle is placed in a superficial vein in the scalp, arm, or leg and connected by a stopcock to two 3-cc syringes filled with bacteriostatic normal saline. For the contrast injection, 0.5 to 3 cc of saline are rapidly injected with a force similar to that of a good hand angiogram from the first syringe followed by a similar injection from the second syringe.*

DETECTION OF RIGHT-TO-LEFT SHUNTS

The microbubbles that give rise to the contrast echoes are filtered completely by the pulmonary and systemic capillary beds. Normally, contrast echoes will not appear in the left heart following a peripheral venous injection. The appearance of contrast echoes in the left heart indicates a right-to-left shunt, either intracardiac or intrapulmonary. Intrapulmonary shunts can be differentiated from intracardiac shunts by the delayed appearance (delay of three to four cardiac cycles) of contrast echoes in the left atrium in intrapulmonary right-to-left shunts.[12] Several investigators have shown that contrast echocardiography is sensitive enough to detect intracardiac right-to-left shunts as small as 5 percent of systemic blood flow.[3,5]

The apical four-chamber view, which images all four cardiac chambers and the atrial and ventricular septa simultaneously, is especially useful for localization of the site of an intracardiac shunt. In patients with atrial right-to-left shunts (Fig. 4-2), contrast echoes first appear in the right atrium and then cross the interatrial septum into the left atrium during rapid ventricular filling and at the onset of ventricular contraction.[5,6] Contrast echoes then enter the right and left ventricles nearly simultaneously by passing through the atrioventricular valve orifices in diastole. This flow pattern can be observed in forms of congenital heart disease with obligatory right-to-left atrial shunting, such as total anomalous pulmonary venous return. Atrial right-to-left shunting is also commonly found in infants with persistent fetal circulation, patients with Ebstein's anomaly of the tricuspid valve, and patients with baffle leaks after Mustard's procedure. In addition, most simple atrial septal defects exhibit bidirectional shunting because of the right-to-left pressure gradient present with the onset of ventricular contraction.[13] Contrast echocardiography is extremely sensitive and can detect this interatrial right-to-left shunt even when systemic arterial saturations are normal and standard dye curves show no right-to-left shunting.[5] The detection of the right-to-left shunt in a simple atrial septal defect can be enhanced by having the patient perform a Valsalva maneuver during the contrast injection. Also, because of streaming, inferior vena caval injections may be more successful in demonstrating the bidirectional flow pattern of an interatrial communication.

In patients with ventricular right-to-left shunts (Fig. 4-3), contrast echoes appear initially in the right atrium and right ventricle and then pass into the left ventricle. The right-to-left ventricular shunt commences with the onset of the isovolumic relaxation phase of ventricular diastole.[5-7] Right-to-left ventricular shunts occur in patients with tetralogy of Fallot, double outlet right ventricle, pulmonary atresia with a ventricular septal defect, and truncus arteriosus. Also, in isolated ventricular septal defects in which the right ventricular pressure is elevated to approximately 50 percent or more of the left ventricular pressure, right-to-left shunting occurs during the isovolumic relaxation phase because of asynchronous changes in pressure of the two ventricles.[6-8,14] In small ventricular septal defects, right ventricular pressure does

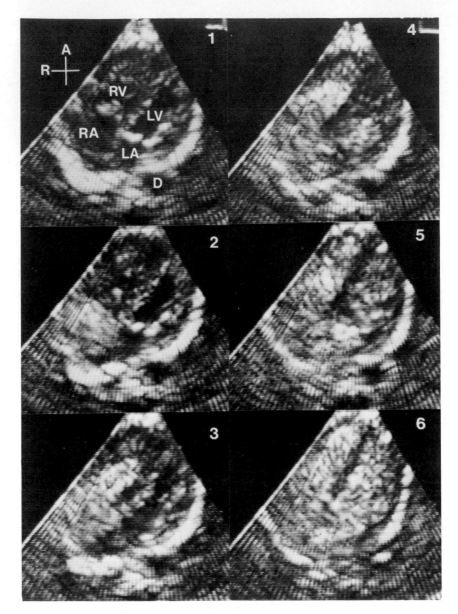

FIG. 4-2. *Peripheral venous contrast injection in the apical four-chamber view from an infant with a right-to-left atrial shunt.* **1.** *Apical four-chamber view prior to the contrast injection. A, apex; D, descending aorta; LA, left atrium; LV, left ventricle; R, right; RA, right atrium; RV, right ventricle.* **2.** *Contrast echoes are filling the RA.* **3.** *Contrast echoes have passed from the RA into the RV. A few contrast echoes have passed across the atrial septum into the LA. The LV and descending aorta are free of contrast echoes.* **4.** *and* **5.** *Contrast echoes have passed across the atrial septum into the LA and subsequently into the LV. The intact ventricular septum is outlined by the contrast echoes filling the two ventricles. The descending aorta is still free of contrast echoes.* **6.** *All four cardiac chambers and the descending aorta are filled with contrast echoes.*

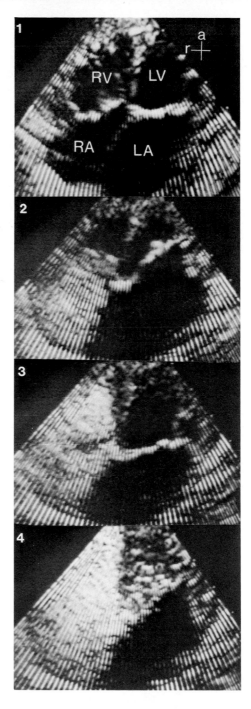

FIG. 4-3. *Peripheral venous contrast injection in the apical four-chamber view from an infant with a large membranous ventricular septal defect.* **1.** *Apical four-chamber view prior to contrast injection. The apical four-chamber view passes through the inlet septum, posterior to the area of the membranous septum. Therefore, the ventricular septal defect in this patient is not seen in this plane. The large left atrium (LA) is indirect evidence of a large left-to-right shunt and increased pulmonary blood flow. a, apex; LV, left ventricle; r, right; RA, right atrium; RV, right ventricle.* **2.** *Contrast echoes are filling the RA.* **3.** *The RV is filled by forward flow of contrast echoes from the RA.* **4.** *Contrast echoes have passed from RV to LV during early diastole. The LA remains free of contrast echoes.*

not exceed left ventricular pressure in early diastole and no right-to-left shunt is seen. In patients with a moderate ventricular septal defect and moderate elevation of the right ventricular pressure, the right-to-left shunt occurs only in early diastole and is transient; however, in patients with near systemic right ventricular pressure and a large ventricular septal defect, the right-to-left shunt occurs throughout the entire duration of diastole.[14] In some patients with systemic pressures in the right ventricle, right-to-left shunting also occurs in late ventricular systole, and blood flows directly from the right ventricle into the aorta. In these patients, contrast echoes arrive during systole in the aorta prior to their filling the left ventricle in diastole (Fig. 4-4).

In patients with right-to-left shunting at both atrial and ventricular levels, a wide variety of contrast echocardiographic flow patterns can occur depending on hemodynamic factors such as the relative sizes of the two defects.[6,15] With a large atrial shunt and a small ventricular shunt, a dense cloud of contrast echoes passes into the left atrium and across the mitral valve, obscuring additional ventricular shunting. With a small atrial shunt and a large ventricular shunt (Fig. 4-5), the area of the mitral valve is poorly opacified, thus allowing direct visualization of both right-to-left shunts.

STRUCTURE IDENTIFICATION

Contrast echocardiography has been especially useful in verifying normal and abnormal anatomic structures seen during the two-dimensional echocardiographic examination. For example, in order to identify certain structures imaged by suprasternal notch echocardiography, a contrast injection was given during cardiac catheterization through a catheter positioned in the right innominate vein (Fig. 4-6). The appearance of a cloud of echoes in the structures along the right side of the transverse aorta identified these structures as the right innominate vein and superior vena cava.

The identity of abnormal cardiac structures can be substantiated by two-dimensional contrast echocardiography. For example, Figures 4-7, 4-8, and 4-9 show a large structure in several echocardiographic planes lying in the area of the atrioventricular groove. This structure was believed to be an abnormal coronary sinus, probably enlarged because of its connection to a persistent left superior vena cava. Echoes from a left arm vein contrast injection first opacified the structure thought to be the coronary sinus and then appeared in the right atrium and right ventricle. Thus, the existence of a persistent left superior vena cava draining to the coronary sinus was verified.[16]

Figure 4-10A is a parasternal short-axis view showing an abnormal cardiac structure believed to be a sinus of Valsalva aneurysm protruding into the right ventricular outflow tract. In Figure 4-10B, contrast echoes from a peripheral venous injection opacify the right heart and outline the abnormal protruding structure. The aortic root and protruding structure are both free of contrast echoes and are, therefore, connected. The suspected identity of the structure was thus confirmed.

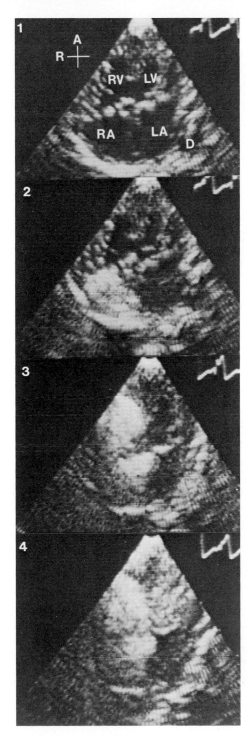

FIG. 4-4. *Peripheral venous contrast injection in the apical four-chamber view from a patient with a large membranous ventricular septal defect and systemic right ventricular pressure.* **1.** *Apical four-chamber view prior to contrast injection. The transducer is tilted slightly anteriorly to visualize the ventricular septal defect. A, apex; D, descending aorta; LA, left atrium; LV, left ventricle; R, right; RA, right atrium; RV, right ventricle.* **2.** *Contrast echoes are filling the RA.* **3.** *Contrast echoes have passed forward from RA to RV. The descending aorta is opacified by contrast echoes that passed from RV to the aorta during late ventricular systole.* **4.** *The body of the LV is filled with contrast echoes that passed from RV to LV during early diastole. The LA remains free of contrast echoes.*

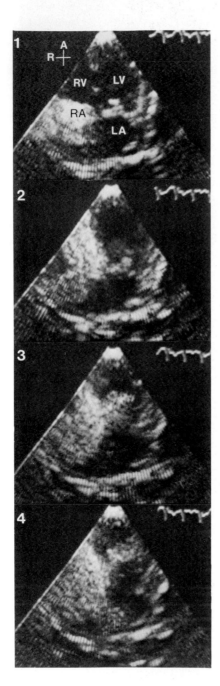

FIG. 4-5. *Peripheral venous contrast injection in the apical four-chamber view from a patient with right-to-left shunting through a large ventricular septal defect and an atrial septal defect.* **1.** *Contrast echoes are filling the right atrium (RA). A, apex; LA, left atrium; LV, left ventricle; R, right; RV, right ventricle.* **2.** *Contrast echoes are filling the RV because of forward flow from the RA.* **3.** *During early diastole, contrast echoes have passed from RV to LV across the ventricular septal defect. The LA is free of contrast echoes.* **4.** *Contrast echoes have now passed from RA to LA across an additional atrial septal defect.*

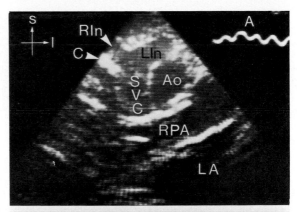

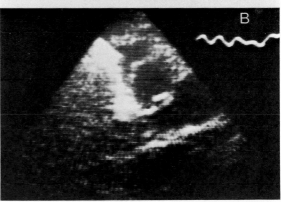

FIG. 4-6. *Contrast injection made during cardiac catheterization in the suprasternal notch short-axis view.* **A.** *A catheter (C) was placed in the right innominate vein (RIn) under fluoroscopy. Ao, aorta; l, left; LA, left atrium; RPA, right pulmonary artery; S, superior; SVC, superior vena cava.* **B.** *During the contrast injection, contrast echoes fill the two structures along the right side of the Ao, confirming that these structures are the right innominate vein and superior vena cava.*

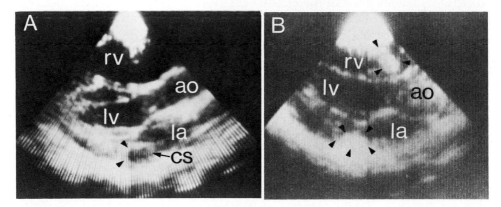

FIG. 4-7. A. *Parasternal long-axis view from a patient with an enlarged coronary sinus (CS) seen in cross section in the atrioventricular groove. A left superior vena cava draining to the coronary sinus was suspected. ao, aorta; la, left atrium; lv, left ventricle; rv, right ventricle.* **B.** *A contrast injection into a left arm vein filled the coronary sinus first and, subsequently, filled the right ventricle. This confirmed the existence of a left superior vena cava draining to the coronary sinus.*

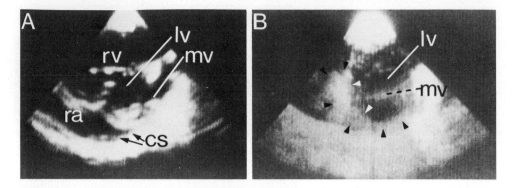

FIG. 4-8. A. *Parasternal short-axis view from a patient with an enlarged coronary sinus (cs). The coronary sinus is seen in tangential section in the atrioventricular groove in this view. lv, left ventricle; mv, mitral valve; ra, right atrium; rv, right ventricle.* **B.** *During a left-arm vein contrast injection, contrast echoes are seen traveling in the coronary sinus toward the right atrium. The contrast echocardiogram verified the existence of a left superior vena cava draining to the coronary sinus.*

Figure 4-11 is a coronal plane through the head of a cyanotic newborn infant. A large circular structure is seen inferior to the lateral ventricles. In order to determine whether this structure was a cystic malformation or a vascular malformation, a peripheral venous contrast injection was made (Fig. 4-11, middle). Contrast echoes that passed from right-to-left at atrial level traveled in the ascending aorta to the carotid arteries and opacified the circular structure. Opacification of the circular structure by contrast echoes confirmed its vascular nature and also confirmed the diagnosis of intracranial arteriovenous malformation.

DEFINITION OF FLOW PATTERNS

After a contrast injection, microbubbles follow the downstream passage of blood and allow the identification of specific flow patterns in certain complex congenital heart defects. Thus, contrast echocardiography adds important physiologic flow information to the anatomic information already obtained from the two-dimensional echocardiogram.[15,17] The following examples show the identification by two-dimensional contrast echocardiography of characteristic flow patterns in several types of heart disease.

In infants with aortic atresia, the ascending aorta, coronary arteries, and vessels to the head and neck are perfused retrograde from the descending aorta by way of a patent ductus arteriosus. Figure 4-12 (top) is a parasternal short-axis view from a patient with aortic atresia prior to a contrast injection. In Figure 4-12 (middle), a contrast injection is made into an umbilical artery catheter positioned in the descending thoracic aorta. The main pulmonary ar-

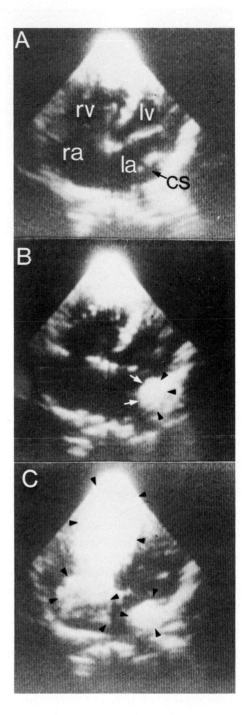

FIG. 4-9. A. *Apical four-chamber view from a patient with tetralogy of Fallot and an enlarged coronary sinus (cs). The right ventricle (rv) is apex forming. A large ventricular septal defect is seen. la, left atrium; lv, left ventricle; ra, right atrium.* **B.** *A left-arm vein contrast injection is made. The coronary sinus fills first with contrast echoes.* **C.** *The right atrium and right ventricle are filled with contrast echoes due to forward flow from the coronary sinus. Subsequent frames showed a right-to-left ventricular shunt. The contrast injection confirmed the presence of a left superior vena cava draining to the coronary sinus.*

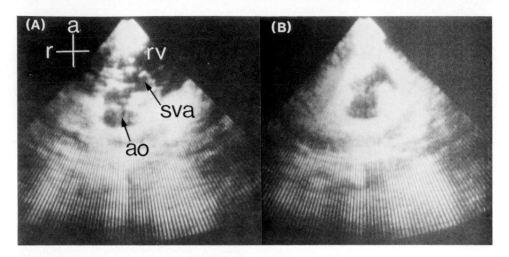

FIG. 4-10. A. *Parasternal short-axis view from a patient with a sinus of Valsalva aneurysm (sva) protruding into the right ventricle (rv). a, anterior; ao, aorta; r, right.* **B.** *During a peripheral venous contrast injection, contrast echoes fill the right ventricle and outline the sinus of Valsalva aneurysm. The sinus of Valsalva aneurysm and the aorta are free of contrast echoes and are connected.*

tery is completely filled by contrast echoes that arrived by way of the patent ductus arteriosus. Finally (Fig. 4-12, bottom), the ascending aorta is filled with contrast echoes that passed retrograde from the descending aorta.

In critically ill newborn infants with a large intracranial arteriovenous fistula, there is usually right-to-left shunting through the foramen ovale and patent ductus arteriosus. Blood passing from right-to-left at the atrial level travels in the systemic circulation to the arteriovenous fistula. In the fistula, blood bypasses the systemic capillary bed and reappears rapidly in the superior vena cava. This specific pattern of early superior vena cava recirculation can be identified by suprasternal notch contrast echocardiography (Fig. 4-13).

Contrast echocardiography is useful not only for identifying intracardiac blood flow patterns but also for defining systemic venous flow patterns. Figure 4-14 (left) is an apical four-chamber view from a patient with polysplenia syndrome and a common atrium. Following a right-arm vein injection (middle), contrast echoes appear in the right-sided atrium. Following a left-arm vein injection (right), contrast echoes appear immediately in the left-sided atrium. These contrast injections confirm the existence of bilateral superior venae cavae draining directly to the right and left side of the common atrium.

In patients who have undergone Mustard's procedure for transposition of the great arteries, contrast echocardiography can be used to detect superior vena caval obstruction. During an arm vein injection in patients with complete superior vena caval obstruction (Fig. 4-15), contrast echoes are seen in

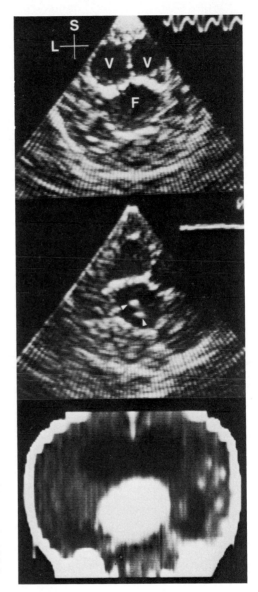

FIG. 4-11. Top. *Two-dimensional sector scan of the brain in the coronal plane from a critically ill newborn infant with a suspected arteriovenous malformation. A large structure is seen inferior to the lateral ventricles (V). F, fistula; L, left; S, superior.* **Middle.** *Following a peripheral venous contrast injection, contrast echoes (arrows) that passed from right-to-left through a patent foramen ovale travel in the systemic circulation and enter the fistula. The appearance of contrast echoes in the structure inferior to the ventricles proves that this structure is a vascular abnormality rather than a cystic malformation.* **Bottom.** *Computerized tomography scan with contrast in the coronal plane for comparison.*

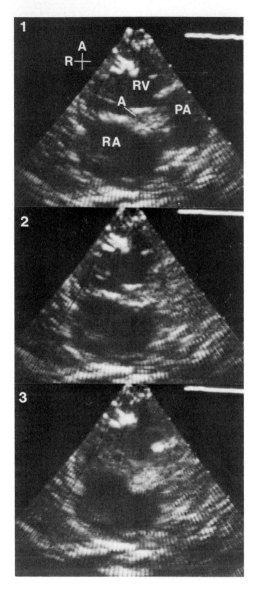

FIG. 4-12. *Contrast echocardiogram in an infant with aortic atresia.* **1.** *Parasternal short-axis view prior to contrast injection. The lumen of the ascending aorta (A) is extremely small. The right atrium (RA), right ventricle (RV), and pulmonary artery (PA) are enlarged. A, anterior; R, right.* **2.** *A contrast injection is given through an umbilical artery catheter positioned in the descending thoracic aorta. Contrast echoes that passed from left-to-right through a patent ductus arteriosus are filling the PA. The aorta is free of contrast echoes.* **3.** *Following their appearance in the PA, contrast echoes are then seen filling the aorta retrograde from the descending aorta injection. Retrograde filling of the ascending aorta, coronary arteries, and vessels to the head and neck is a characteristic flow pattern in infants with hypoplastic left heart complex.*

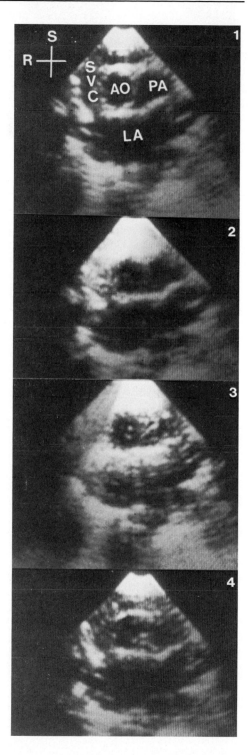

FIG. 4-13. *Peripheral venous contrast injection in an infant with an intracranial arteriovenous malformation to show the pattern of early superior vena cava recirculation present in patients with this abnormality.* **1.** *Suprasternal notch short-axis view prior to contrast injection. AO, aorta; LA, left atrium; PA, pulmonary artery; R, right; S, superior; SVC, superior vena cava.* **2.** *Contrast echoes from an arm vein injection are filling the SVC.* **3.** *Contrast echoes are seen in the LA, PA, and AO because of a right-to-left shunt through the patent foramen ovale.* **4.** *The AO, PA, and LA are relatively free of echoes from the contrast injection; however, contrast echoes have reappeared in the SVC. The SVC recirculation is caused by contrast passing from left-to-right through the intracranial arteriovenous malformation.*

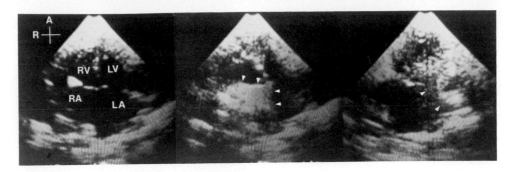

FIG. 4-14. Left. *Apical four-chamber view from a patient with polysplenia syndrome and a common atrium. A, apex; LA, left-sided atrium; LV, left ventricle; R, right; RA, right-sided atrium; RV, right ventricle.* **Middle.** *A contrast injection into a right arm vein fills the RA, confirming the presence of a right superior vena cava draining to the RA.* **Right.** *A contrast injection into a left arm vein fills the LA confirming the presence of a left superior vena cava draining directly to the LA.*

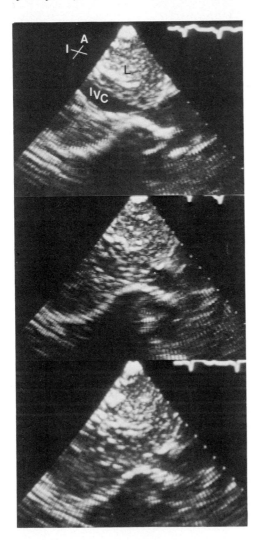

FIG. 4-15. *Contrast echocardiogram in the subcostal long-axis view from a patient with total superior vena caval obstruction following Mustard's procedure.* **Top.** *The junction of the inferior vena cava (IVC) and systemic venous atrium is seen prior to the contrast injection. A, anterior; I, inferior; L, liver.* **Middle.** *Contrast echoes are seen in the lower IVC traveling toward the heart. The systemic venous atrium is free of contrast echoes.* **Bottom.** *The entire IVC is filled with contrast echoes arriving by way of azygous–IVC collateral vessels.*

the inferior vena cava traveling toward the systemic venous atrium. These contrast echoes arrive in the inferior vena cava by way of azygous collateral circulation.

DETECTION OF LEFT-TO-RIGHT SHUNTS

Left-to-right shunts can be diagnosed at cardiac catheterization by contrast injections made into the left heart. Some types of left-to-right shunt can also be detected by peripheral venous contrast echocardiography. During contrast injections in patients with an atrial septal defect, noncontrast-containing blood passes across the atrial septum and washes contrast-containing blood out of the right atrium. This left-to-right atrial shunt produces a negative contrast effect in the right atrium (Fig. 4-16).[18]

Left-to-right shunting through a patent ductus arteriosus can be detected by contrast injections into an umbilical artery catheter positioned in the descending thoracic aorta. Opacification of the transverse aorta and pulmonary artery during the contrast echocardiogram confirms a ductal left-to-right shunt.[17] In patients with a large left-to-right ductal shunt, contrast echoes can often be seen passing forwards and backwards in the descending abdominal aorta by using the subcostal long-axis view. This flow pattern is caused by diastolic run-off from the descending aorta in patients with a large patent ductus arteriosus.

SPONTANEOUS MICROCAVITATIONS

During the two-dimensional echocardiographic examination in some patients who do not have an indwelling venous line, spontaneous contrast echoes can be seen passing through the systemic veins and right heart. Spontaneous microcavitations are seen most often in patients with impaired forward flow in the right heart (Fig. 4-17), hemodynamically significant pericardial effusions (Fig. 4-18), or severe congestive heart failure. Similarly, spontaneous microcavitations have been seen in the left heart, especially in patients with artificial valves.[13] The origin and significance of spontaneous microcavitations is unclear at present. Spontaneous microcavitations observed at echocardiography in patients with and without indwelling venous lines and at cardiac catheterization during indocyanine dye injections lead us to believe that contrast echocardiography is a benign procedure.

SUMMARY

Contrast echocardiography was initially used to verify cardiac anatomy. Since its early use, this technique has become invaluable for detecting right-to-left

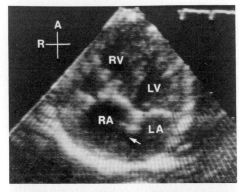

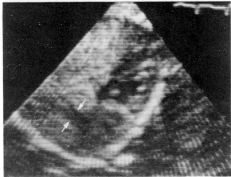

FIG. 4-16. Top. *Apical four-chamber view prior to contrast injection from a patient with a secundum atrial septal defect (arrow). The right atrium (RA) and right ventricle (RV) are dilated because of the large left-to-right atrial shunt. A, apex; LA, left atrium; LV, left ventricle; R, right.* **Bottom.** *Following a peripheral venous contrast injection, the right atrium and right ventricle are filled with contrast echoes. A jet of noncontrast-containing blood has passed from left-to-right across the atrial septal defect and washed contrast-containing blood out of the right atrium (arrows). This creates a negative contrast effect in the right atrium.*

shunts, left-to-right shunts, and specific flow patterns characteristic of certain complex congenital heart defects. Contrast echocardiography adds important physiologic information to the anatomic study of the heart by the two-dimensional sector scan.

FIG. 4-17. *Subcostal long-axis view of the inferior vena cava (IVC) from a patient with severe congestive heart failure following Fontan's procedure for tricuspid atresia. Spontaneous microcavitations (arrows) are seen in the hepatic veins (H). The patient did not have an indwelling venous line. A, anterior; I, inferior.*

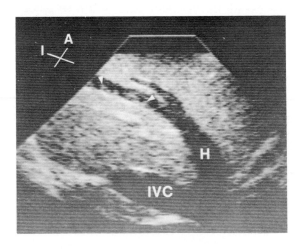

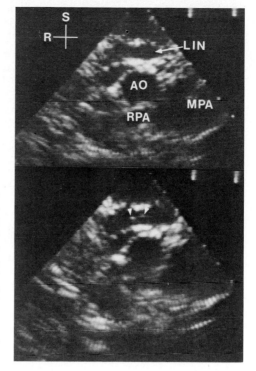

FIG. 4-18. Top. *Suprasternal notch short-axis view from a patient with a hemodynamically significant pericardial effusion following a pulmonary valvotomy. There is poststenotic dilatation of the main pulmonary artery (MPA). AO, aorta; LIN, left innominate vein; R, right; RPA, right pulmonary artery; S, superior.* **Bottom.** *Although the patient had no indwelling venous line, spontaneous microcavitations (arrows) appeared in the innominate veins throughout the echocardiographic study.*

REFERENCES

1. Gramiak R, Shah PM: Echocardiography of the aortic root. Invest Radiol 3: 356, 1968
2. Gramiak R, Shah PM, Kramer DH: Ultrasound cardiography: Contrast studies in anatomy and function. Radiology 92: 939, 1969
3. Pieroni DR, Varghese PJ, Freedom RM, Rowe RD: The sensitivity of contrast echocardiography in detecting intracardiac shunts. Cathet Cardiovasc Diagn 5: 19, 1979
4. Kerber RE, Kioschos JM, Lauer RM: Use of an ultrasonic contrast method in the diagnosis of valvular regurgitation and intracardiac shunts. Am J Cardiol 34: 722, 1974
5. Seward JB, Tajik AJ, Spangler JG, Ritter DG: Echocardiographic contrast studies: initial experience. Mayo Clin Proc 50: 163, 1975
6. Valdes-Cruz LM, Pieroni DR, Roland J-MA, Varghese PJ: Echocardiographic detection of intracardiac right-to-left shunts following peripheral vein injections. Circulation 54: 558, 1976
7. Seward JB, Tajik AJ, Hagler DJ, Ritter DG: Peripheral venous contrast echocardiography. Am J Cardiol 39: 202, 1977
8. Serruys PW, van den Brand M, Hugenholtz PG, Roelandt J: Intracardiac right-to-

left shunts demonstrated by two-dimensional echocardiography after peripheral vein injection. Br Heart J 42: 429, 1979

9. Kremkau FW, Gramiak R, Carstensen EL, Shah PM, Kramer DH: Ultrasonic detection of cavitation at catheter tips. Am J Roentgenol 110: 177, 1970

10. Barrera JG, Fulkerson PK, Rittgers SE, Nerem RM: The nature of contrast echocardiographic targets. Circulation (Suppl II) 57–58: II-233, 1978 (abstract)

11. Meltzer RS, Tickner EG, Sahines TP, Popp RL: The source of ultrasound contrast effect. J Clin Ultrasound 8: 121, 1980

12. Shub C, Tajik AJ, Seward JB, Dines DE: Detecting intrapulmonary right-to-left shunt with contrast echocardiography: Observations in a patient with diffuse pulmonary arteriovenous fistulas. Mayo Clin Proc 51: 81, 1976

13. Fraker TD Jr, Harris PJ, Behar VS, Kisslo JA: Detection and exclusion of interatrial shunts by two-dimensional echocardiography and peripheral venous injection. Circulation 59: 379, 1979

14. Serwer GA, Armstrong BE, Anderson PAW, Sherman D, Benson DW Jr, Edwards SB: Use of contrast echocardiography for evaluation of right ventricular hemodynamics in the presence of ventricular septal defects. Circulation 58: 327, 1978

15. Tajik AJ, Seward JB: Contrast echocardiography. Cardiovasc Clin 9: 317, 1978

16. Snider AR, Ports TA, Silverman NH: Venous anomalies of the coronary sinus: Detection by M-mode, two-dimensional and contrast echocardiography. Circulation 60: 721, 1979

17. Sahn DJ, Allen HD, George W, Mason M, Goldberg SJ: The utility of contrast echocardiographic techniques in the care of critically ill infants with cardiac and pulmonary disease. Circulation 56: 959, 1977

18. Weyman AE, Wann LS, Caldwell RL, Hurwitz RA, Dillon JC, Feigenbaum H: Negative contrast echocardiography: A new method for detecting left-to-right shunts. Circulation 59: 498, 1979

CHAPTER 5

Left-to-Right Shunts

ATRIAL SEPTAL DEFECT

Atrial septal defects are a common cause of left-to-right intracardiac shunting. These defects may occur in the lower portion of the atrial septum adjacent to the atrioventricular valves (ostium primum defects), in the midportion of the atrial septum (ostium secundum defects), or in the superior portion of the atrial septum near its junction with the superior vena cava (sinus venosus defects). Most large atrial septal defects cause right ventricular volume overload, which is manifested on the M-mode echocardiographic examination as an increased right ventricular diastolic dimension and abnormal interventricular septal motion.[1-5] Two-dimensional echocardiography has been a valuable technique for differentiating atrial septal defects from other causes of right ventricular volume overload.[6-9] The following sections describe the two-dimensional echocardiographic features of atrial septal defects. Ostium primum atrial septal defects will be discussed separately in the section on atrioventricular canal defects.

Chamber Size

Most atrial septal defects with significant left-to-right atrial shunting cause enlargement of the right atrium, right ventricle, and pulmonary arteries (Fig. 5-1). Enlargement of the right atrium and right ventricle is most apparent in the apical and subcostal four-chamber views and in the parasternal and subcostal short-axis views. Pulmonary artery enlargement can be seen by suprasternal notch echocardiography. Since the development of pulmonary hyper-

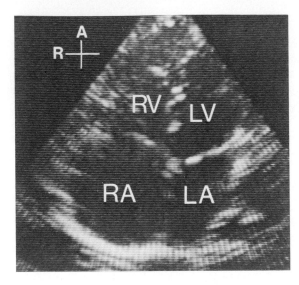

FIG. 5-1. *Apical four-chamber view from a patient with a large secundum atrial septal defect. The right atrium (RA) and right ventricle (RV) are enlarged. The RV is apex forming. An area of echocardiographic dropout is present in the midportion of the interatrial septum. A, apex; LA, left atrium; LV, left ventricle; R, right.*

tension in isolated atrial septal defects is uncommon in childhood, the right ventricular anterior wall is of normal thickness in these views.

As the right ventricle enlarges into the left chest, the left ventricle is pushed posteriorly and laterally. This clockwise rotation of the entire heart by the dilated right ventricle with resultant posterior displacement of the apical impulse may lead to difficulty in obtaining the apical views. The apex can be made more accessible by having the patient lie in the left lateral decubitus position over a large semicircular hole cut out off the edge of the mattress. In the apical four-chamber view, the enlarged right ventricle often occupies most of the cardiac apex (Fig. 5-1).

Right ventricular volume overload causes vigorous right ventricular ejection that can be seen in the parasternal and subcostal short-axis views through the base of the heart. In these views, a hyperdynamic, to-and-fro motion of the right ventricular outflow tract can be seen. The vigorous pulsation of the main pulmonary artery, which can be seen in the short-axis and suprasternal notch views, is the echocardiographic equivalent of the radiographic "hilar dance."

In some patients with a small atrial septal defect, the right atrium and right ventricle are of normal size. Right atrial and right ventricular enlargement caused by an atrial septal defect may be difficult to distinguish from the normal pattern of right heart dominance seen in newborn infants.

In patients with an atrial septal defect, the left atrial size is usually normal. If the left atrium is enlarged, additional defects should be suspected.

Abnormal Septal Motion

In the normal heart, the ventricular septum at the level of the posterior mitral valve leaflet or below moves posteriorly in systole. In conditions causing right ventricular enlargement, this portion of the ventricular septum moves anteriorly in systole. Systolic anterior septal motion or paradoxical septal motion occurs in defects such as atrial septal defect, anomalous pulmonary venous return, tricuspid and pulmonary insufficiency, Ebstein's anomaly, and in patients with ventricular septal patches.[3–5,10] Using parasternal short-axis views, Weyman and colleagues showed that paradoxical septal motion is caused by a change in the diastolic shape of the left ventricle.[11] In the parasternal short-axis view at the level of the posterior mitral valve leaflet in normal patients, the left ventricle is circular in systole and diastole. In systole, the septum and right ventricular anterior wall move toward the left ventricular posterior wall. In the parasternal short-axis view of patients with right ventricular enlargement, the septum is flattened in diastole or has a totally reversed curvature (Fig. 5-2). As the septum moves anteriorly in systole, the left ventricle resumes its normal circular configuration. Paradoxical septal motion also occurs in the parasternal long-axis view and the apical four-chamber view.

In patients with a small atrial septal defect or associated lesions, the ventricular septal motion may be normal. Also, because of right heart dominance at birth, flattened ventricular septal motion can occur normally in newborn infants. It is important to note that the upper portion of the ventricular septum near the aortic root normally moves anteriorly in systole.

Direct Visualization of Defects

Secundum atrial septal defects can be visualized directly by two-dimensional echocardiography as an area of echocardiographic dropout in the midportion

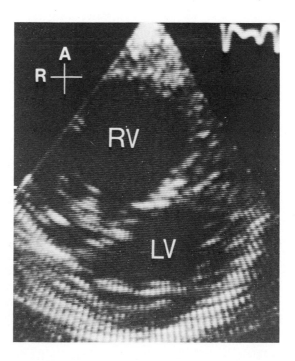

FIG. 5-2. *Parasternal short-axis view through the left ventricle (LV) from a patient with right ventricular volume overload. Because of the large right ventricle (RV), the septum has a reversed curvature in diastole. A, anterior; R, right.*

of the interatrial septum (Fig. 5-1). The apical and subcostal four-chamber views and the parasternal and subcostal short-axis views are most useful for imaging atrial septal defects. In most patients with atrial septal defects, echocardiographic dropout can be seen in the interatrial septum; however, in many normal patients, echocardiographic dropout can be seen in the same area because of the thinness of the fossa ovalis.[12] Thus, it is unwise to diagnose a secundum atrial septal defect on the basis of echocardiographic dropout alone.

Peripheral venous contrast echocardiography is useful for distinguishing an atrial septal defect from normal echocardiographic dropout in the area of the fossa ovalis. Most patients with an atrial septal defect have a right-to-left shunt at the onset of ventricular contraction. Right-to-left atrial shunting and the negative contrast effect in patients with atrial septal defect are discussed in detail in Chapter 4.

We have thus far been unsuccessful in directly visualizing sinus venosus defects. In patients who have undergone patch closure of an atrial septal defect, the bright echoes arising from the patch help identify the anatomic location of the previous atrial septal defect (Fig. 5-3).

VENTRICULAR SEPTAL DEFECT

Ventricular septal defects alone or in combination with other lesions account for a large proportion of congenital heart disease. The ventricular septum is a complex structure consisting of several portions with different embryologic derivations. These portions include the membranous septum, the sinus or inlet septum, the trabeculated or muscular septum, and the infundibular or outlet septum (Fig. 5-4A).[13,14] Ventricular septal defects are usually not isolated to a single part of the ventricular septum but occur along fusion lines between the various portions of the ventricular septum. Ventricular septal de-

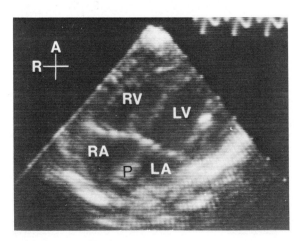

FIG. 5-3. *Apical four-chamber view from a patient who had recently undergone patch closure of a secundum atrial septal defect. The right atrium (RA) and the right ventricle (RV) are still enlarged. The RV is apex forming. The highly reflective dacron patch (P) is seen positioned in the area where secundum atrial septal defects are usually located. A, apex; LA, left atrium; LV, left ventricle; R, right.*

FIG. 5-4. A. *Diagrammatic representation of the parts of the ventricular septum as viewed from the right ventricle (above) and left ventricle (below). Ao, aorta; LA, left atrium; LV, left ventricle; PA, pulmonary artery; RA, right atrium; RV, right ventricle. The figure was provided courtesy of Dr. Robert Anderson.*

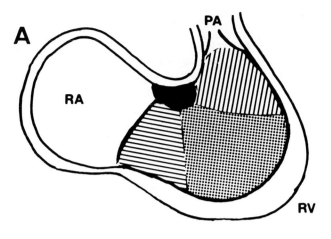

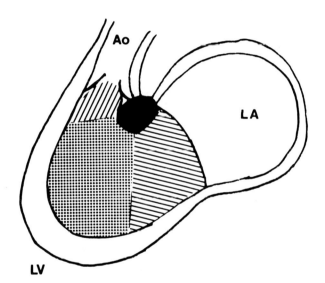

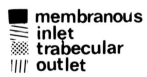
membranous
inlet
trabecular
outlet

fects can be detected by two-dimensional echocardiography[15-21]; however, because of the curvature and complexity of the septum, a variety of echocardiographic planes is necessary for complete examination of each portion of the ventricular septum (Fig. 5-4B).

Chamber Size

In patients with moderate or large ventricular septal defects and normal pulmonary vascular resistances, the increased pulmonary blood flow and in-

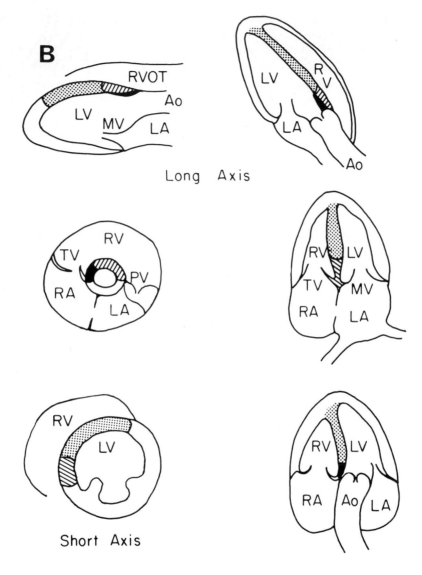

FIG. 5-4. B. *Diagrammatic representation of the parts of the ventricular septum seen in the long-axis, short-axis, and four-chamber views. This figure was drawn after the diagrams of Dr. G. Van Mill.*[19]

creased pulmonary venous return cause dilatation of the left atrium and left ventricle.[22–24] This left heart enlargement can be seen in the parasternal and apical long-axis views and in the apical and subcostal four-chamber views. In the four-chamber views, the atrial septum bulges toward the right. Because of the volume overload, the left ventricular stroke volume is increased. Exaggerated septal and left ventricular posterior wall motion is observed in the parasternal, apical, and subcostal views. These signs of left ventricular volume overload are not specific for ventricular septal defects but can be seen in other defects causing left ventricular volume overload such as patent ductus arteriosus and aortic and mitral insufficiency.

In patients with isolated ventricular septal defects and normal pulmonary vascular resistances, the right ventricular anterior wall and left ventricular posterior wall are of normal thickness. In patients with isolated ventricular septal defects and elevated pulmonary vascular resistances, the left atrium and left ventricle are often of normal size and the right ventricular anterior wall thickness is increased.

Direct Visualization of the Defect

Ventricular septal defects can be imaged directly as areas of echocardiographic dropout in the ventricular septum. To avoid false positive diagnoses, the echocardiographic dropout should be seen in at least two planes. Often, the edges of the ventricular septum that border the defect are unusually bright and create the appearance of a T on the two-dimensional echocardiogram. It is believed that the edges of the ventricular septal defect act as specular reflectors of ultrasound and give rise to the T artifact.[18]

Membranous Ventricular Septal Defects. Membranous ventricular septal defects are located in a superior, subaortic portion of the ventricular septum beneath the septal leaflet of the tricuspid valve (Fig. 5-4). Most large membranous ventricular septal defects can be imaged in the parasternal and apical long-axis views as an absence of echoes between the septum and anterior aortic root (Fig. 5-5). Large membranous defects can be distinguished from infundibular defects (which occur in the same area of the septum in the apical and parasternal long-axis views) by the absence of override of the ventricular sep-

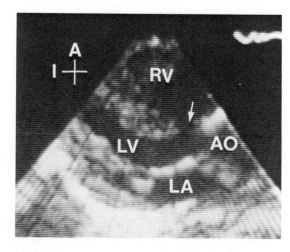

FIG. 5-5. *Parasternal long-axis view from an infant with a large membranous ventricular septal defect (arrow). The defect is located in the superior portion of the ventricular septum just beneath the aortic valve. A, anterior; AO, aorta; I, inferior; LA, left atrium; LV, left ventricle; RV, right ventricle.*

tum by the aorta. In order to visualize most membranous defects in the parasternal and apical long-axis views, it is necessary to examine the septum between the aortic and tricuspid valves by orienting the plane toward the right.

In order to visualize membranous defects in the parasternal and subcostal short-axis views, the transducer is oriented from the apex to the base of the heart in a transverse plane. Just beneath the aortic valve in the short-axis view, membranous defects can be visualized in the septum adjacent to the tricuspid valve (Fig. 5-6).

In the apical and subcostal four-chamber views, the transducer must be oriented cranially toward the aortic root in order to visualize the area of the membranous ventricular septum (Figs. 5-7 and 5-8). Unless they are very large, membranous defects cannot be seen in the standard four-chamber views that pass through the inlet septum posterior to the membranous septum.

Recent studies suggest that a large proportion of membranous ventricular septal defects diminish significantly in size or close spontaneously by aneurysm formation.[25-27] Aneurysms of the membranous septum are small, conical projections of thin membrane arising from the margins of ventricular septal defects. On the two-dimensional echocardiogram, ventricular septal aneurysms appear as saccular structures protruding into the right ventricle in systole just beneath the septal leaflet of the tricuspid valve (Figs. 5-9 to 5-12).[28,29] Because of the pressure difference between the right and left ventricles, the aneurysms protrude into the right ventricle in systole and realign with the ventricular septum in diastole. This systolic expansion and diastolic realignment of the septal aneurysm creates a cyclical, flicking motion in real time. Natural history studies and cardiac catheterization data suggest that septal aneurysms are usually associated with a benign, asymptomatic course and favorable hemodynamics ($Q_p/Q_s < 2.0$)[27,29]

Approximately one third of the patients we have studied with an isolated ventricular septal defect have had a ventricular septal aneurysm by M-mode

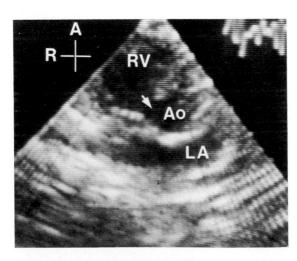

FIG. 5-6. *Parasternal short-axis view from a patient with a large membranous ventricular septal defect (arrow). The defect is located just beneath the aortic valve and adjacent to the septal leaflet of the tricuspid valve. A, anterior; Ao, aorta; LA, left atrium; R, right; RV, right ventricle.*

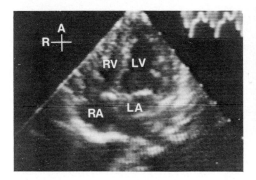 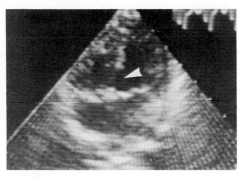

FIG. 5-7. *Apical four-chamber views from a patient with a membranous ventricular septal defect (arrow). The defect is not seen in the standard apical four-chamber view (***Left***) which passes through the inlet septum posterior to the membranous septum. The defect can be seen with cranial angulation of the transducer toward the aortic root from the standard apical four-chamber view (***Right***). A, apex; LA, left atrium; LV, left ventricle; R, right; RA, right atrium; RV, right ventricle.*

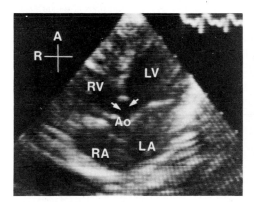 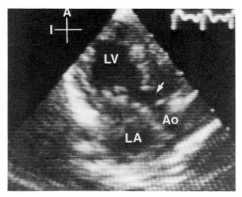

FIG. 5-8. Left. *Apical four-chamber view from a patient with a membranous ventricular septal defect (arrows). The transducer is oriented cranially toward the aortic root in order to visualize the membranous septum. A, apex; Ao, aorta; LA, left atrium; LV, left ventricle; R, right; RA, right atrium; RV, right ventricle.* **Right.** *Apical long-axis view from a patient with a membranous ventricular septal defect (arrow) located in the superior portion of the septum just beneath the aortic valve. A, apex; Ao, aorta; I, inferior; LA, left atrium; LV, left ventricle.*

and/or two-dimensional echocardiography. Because it yields fewer false positive diagnoses, two-dimensional echocardiography is more accurate than M-mode echocardiography for detecting ventricular septal aneurysms. The base of the ventricular septal aneurysm reflects the size of the original defect (Fig. 5-11), and the location of the septal aneurysm identifies the area of the membranous septum. In patients who have undergone patch closure of a

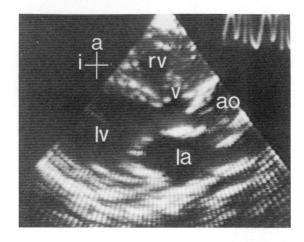

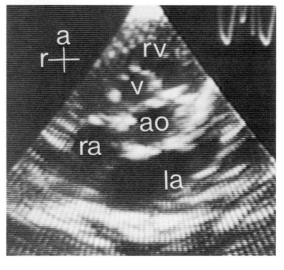

FIG. 5-9. *Parasternal   long-axis view from a patient with a ventricular septal aneurysm (v). The aneurysm appears as a saccular structure protruding into the right ventricle (rv) in systole. a, anterior; ao, aorta; i, inferior; la, left atrium; lv, left ventricle.*

FIG. 5-10. *Parasternal short-axis view from a patient with a membranous ventricular septal defect and a ventricular septal aneurysm (v). The aneurysm is seen protruding into the right ventricle (rv) in systole adjacent to the tricuspid valve septal leaflet. a, anterior; ao, aorta; la, left atrium; r, right; ra, right atrium.*

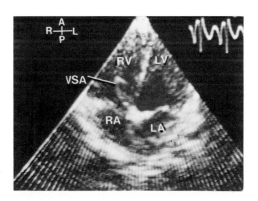

FIG.   5-11. *Apical   four-chamber view from a patient with a membranous ventricular septal defect and a ventricular septal aneurysm (VSA). The aneurysm is protruding into the right ventricle (RV) in systole adjacent to the tricuspid valve. The base of the aneurysm may reflect the size of the original defect. A, anterior; L, left; LA, left atrium; LV, left ventricle; P, posterior; R, right; RA, right atrium.*

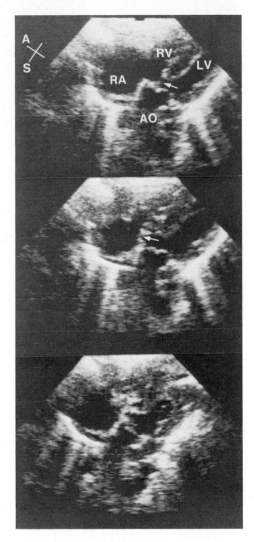

FIG. 5-12. *Subcostal views from a patient with a membranous ventricular septal defect and a ventricular septal aneurysm. In the top frame, the defect is seen (arrow). In the other two frames in systole, the ventricular septal aneurysm is seen protruding into the right ventricle (RV). A, anterior; AO, aorta; LV, left ventricle; RA, right atrium; S, superior.*

membranous ventricular septal defect, the highly reflective patch also provides a marker for the area of the membranous septum (Fig. 5-13).

Muscular Ventricular Septal Defects. Muscular ventricular septal defects are located in the inferior portion of the ventricular septum that extends from beneath the membranous septum to the cardiac apex (Fig. 5-4). Although some of these defects can be imaged directly in the parasternal and apical long-axis views, they are better visualized by examining the trabeculated ventricular septum in cross section from the base to the apex of the heart in the parasternal and subcostal short-axis views (Fig. 5-14). In the apical and subcostal four-chamber views, muscular ventricular septal defects are usually located in the

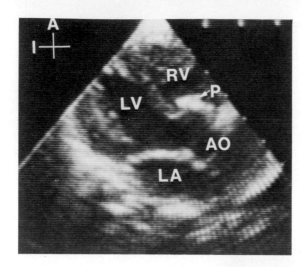

FIG. 5-13. *Parasternal long-axis view from a patient who has undergone patch (P) closure of a membranous ventricular septal defect. Bright echoes are arising from the artificial patch material. The patch is positioned in the area of the membranous septum. A, anterior; AO, aorta; I, inferior; LA, left atrium; LV, left ventricle; RV, right ventricle.*

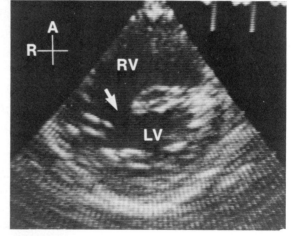

FIG. 5-14. *Parasternal short-axis view through the left ventricle (LV) at the level of the papillary muscles from a patient with a large muscular ventricular septal defect (arrow). The defect is located in the inferior portion of the septum near the cardiac apex. A, anterior; R, right, RV, right ventricle.*

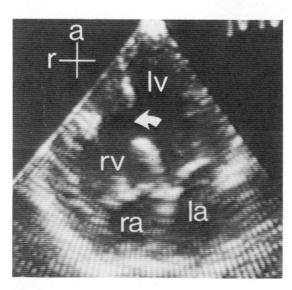

FIG. 5-15. *Apical four-chamber view from an infant with a large muscular ventricular septal defect (arrow). The defect is located in the inferior, trabeculated septum. a, apex; la, left atrium; lv, left ventricle; r, right; ra, right atrium; rv, right ventricle.*

inferior two-thirds of the ventricular septum (Figs. 5-15, 5-16). In patients who have undergone patch closure of a muscular ventricular septal defect, the highly reflective patch provides a marker for the area of the trabeculated septum (Figs. 5-17, 5-18).

Defects in the Inlet Septum. The inlet or sinus portion of the ventricular septum is the posterior part of the septum adjacent to the atrioventricular valves (Fig. 5-4). The atrioventricular canal type of ventricular septal defect and the ventricular septal defect in patients with tricuspid atresia are examples of inlet septal defects. The apical and subcostal four-chamber views, which pass through both atrioventricular valves and the posterior ventricular septum, are

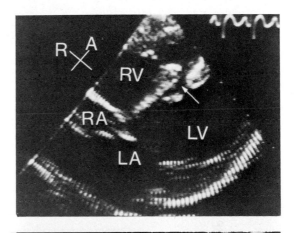

FIG. 5-16. *Subcostal four-chamber view from a child with a traumatic ventricular septal defect (arrow) in the trabeculated septum. The left atrium (LA) and left ventricle (LV) are enlarged. A, apex; R, right; RA, right atrium; RV, right ventricle.*

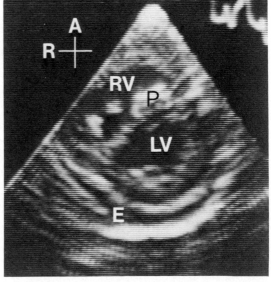

FIG. 5-17. *Parasternal short-axis view through the left ventricle (LV) at the level of the papillary muscles from a patient who had undergone patch (P) closure of a muscular ventricular septal defect. The highly reflective patch is positioned in the inferior portion of the septum near the cardiac apex. The right ventricular anterior wall is thickened due to previous pulmonary hypertension. A small posterior pericardial effusion (E) is present. A, anterior; R, right; RV, right ventricle.*

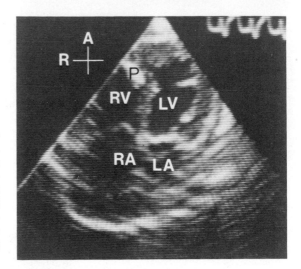

FIG. 5-18. *Apical four-chamber view from a patient who had undergone patch (P) closure of a muscular ventricular septal defect. The highly reflective patch is positioned in the trabeculated ventricular septum near the cardiac apex. A, apex; LA, left atrium; LV, left ventricle; R, right; RA, right atrium; RV, right ventricle.*

most useful for visualizing these defects (Fig. 5-19). In the parasternal and subcostal short-axis views through the left ventricle, inlet defects are situated adjacent to the tricuspid valve but in a plane inferior to that used to visualize the membranous septum (Fig. 5-20).

Infundibular or Conotruncal Ventricular Septal Defects. The outlet or infundibular portion of the ventricular septum is the anterior part of the ventricular septum located just beneath the aortic and pulmonic valves (Fig. 5-4).

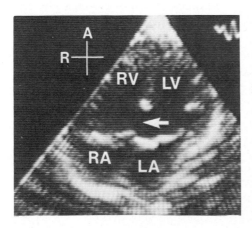
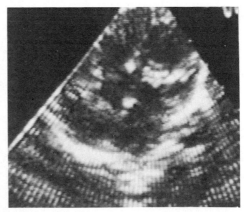

FIG. 5-19. *Apical four-chamber views in systole (**Left**) and diastole (**Right**) from a patient with a ventricular septal defect (arrow) of the atrioventricular canal type located in the inlet septum, which is posterior and adjacent to the atrioventricular valves. The edges of the defect act as specular reflectors of ultrasound and are highly reflective. A, apex; LA, left atrium; LV, left ventricle; R, right; RA, right atrium; RV, right ventricle.*

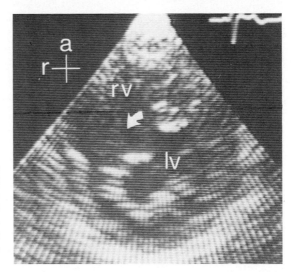

FIG. 5-20. *Parasternal short-axis view through the left ventricle (lv) from a patient with tricuspid atresia and a ventricular septal defect (arrow). The diminutive right ventricle (rv) is seen anteriorly. The defect is located in the inlet septum. a, anterior; r, right.*

Ventricular septal defects in this portion of the septum are called infundibular or conotruncal defects and occur in patients with lesions such as tetralogy of Fallot, truncus arteriosus, and double outlet right ventricle. These defects are usually associated with override of the ventricular septum by the aorta. The parasternal and apical long-axis views, which display the spatial relations between the septum and anterior aortic root, are especially useful for imaging these defects (Figs. 5-21, 5-22). Often, with cranial angulation of the transducer from the standard apical or subcostal four-chamber views, the infundibular defect and aortic–septal malalignment can be seen (Fig. 5-22).

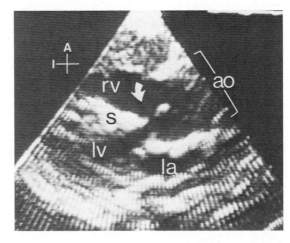

FIG. 5-21. *Parasternal long-axis view from a patient with tetralogy of Fallot. A large ventricular septal defect (arrow) is seen in the infundibular or outlet septum just beneath the aortic valve. The aorta (ao) overrides the ventricular septum (s). Aortic override of the septum is characteristic of conotruncal ventricular septal defects. The right ventricular anterior wall is thickened due to severe pulmonary stenosis. A, anterior; I, inferior; la, left atrium; lv, left ventricle; rv, right ventricle.*

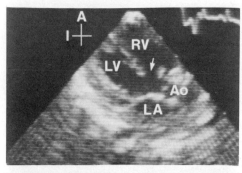

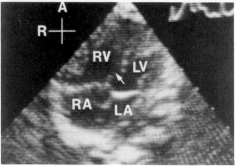

FIG. 5-22. **Top.** *Apical long-axis view from a patient with a conotruncal or malalignment ventricular septal defect (arrow). The defect is located in the anterior portion of the septum beneath the aortic valve. The aorta (Ao) overrides the septum slightly. A, anterior; I, inferior; LA, left atrium; LV, left ventricle; RV, right ventricle.* **Bottom.** *Apical four-chamber view from the same patient. The malalignment ventricular septal defect (arrow) is seen by tilting the transducer cranially. A, apex; LA, left atrium; LV, left ventricle; R, right; RA, right atrium; RV, right ventricle.*

Difficulties in Direct Visualization of Ventricular Septal Defects

The complex curvature of the ventricular septum makes visualization of the entire septum from any one echocardiographic plane impossible and may lead to artifactual dropout in areas where the septum curves out of the echocardiographic plane. For this reason, it is important that an area of echocardiographic dropout be seen in at least two planes before making the diagnosis of ventricular septal defect.

It has been shown that ventricular septal defects are larger in diastole than in systole.[18] The changing size of the ventricular septal defect throughout the cardiac cycle and the overall cardiac motion can make the distinction between a true ventricular septal defect and artifactual echocardiographic dropout difficult. Also, artifactual dropout can occur in the area of the thin membranous septum if gain settings are too low.

The ventricular septum is best visualized when it is perpendicular to the plane of sound. In some echocardiographic planes, portions of the ventricular septum can be parallel to the plane of sound, thus causing artifactual echocardiographic dropout in the septum. Indeed, it is possible for the entire septum to be parallel to the plane of sound in a particular view and create the appearance of a single ventricle (see Chap. 10).

In studies on the ability of two-dimensional echocardiography to detect ventricular septal defects, large defects were detected with a high degree of accuracy; however, small defects were often difficult to resolve.[17-20] Recent in vitro studies have shown that the size of the ventricular septal defect on the two-dimensional image varies with the type of equipment used but is always smaller than the actual defect size.[21]

Contrast Echocardiography

The use of peripheral venous contrast echocardiography to detect a right-to-left shunt at ventricular level was discussed in Chapter 4. Contrast echocardiography is a useful technique for proving a ventricular shunt when the defect cannot be imaged directly with certainty.

ATRIOVENTRICULAR CANAL DEFECT

Lack of fusion of the embryonic endocardial cushion tissue leads to a variety of anatomic defects involving the atrioventricular valves and/or the cardiac septa. In patients with atrioventricular canal defects, M-mode echocardiographic studies have shown a wide spectrum of abnormal findings including abnormal opposition of the septum and anterior mitral valve leaflet in diastole, abnormal mitral valve orientation, and a common atrioventricular valve leaflet crossing the ventricular septum.[30-36] Because it allows estimation of the size of the septal defects and definition of the morphology and attachments of the atrioventricular valve leaflets, two-dimensional echocardiography has been especially useful for diagnosis and classification of the anatomic type of atrioventricular canal defect.[37-41]

Incomplete Atrioventricular Canal Defect

Ostium Primum Atrial Septal Defect. The most common form of incomplete atrioventricular canal defect is the ostium primum atrial septal defect with a cleft anterior mitral valve leaflet. The ostium primum atrial septal defect is imaged best in the apical and subcostal four-chamber views (Figs. 5-23, 5-24). In these views, the lower portion of the atrial septum adjacent to the atrioventricular valves is absent. The atrial septum bordering the ostium primum defect has a bulbous appearance, which gives the remaining atrial septum a matchstick configuration.[40] Frequently, because of associated secundum atrial septal defects or echo dropout in the area of the fossa ovalis, only a bright dot of echoes can be seen arising from the atrial septum that rims the ostium primum defect. Patients with ostium primum atrial septal defects usually have evidence of right atrial and right ventricular enlargement on the four-chamber views. Frequently, right ventricular volume overload with paradoxical septal motion is present.

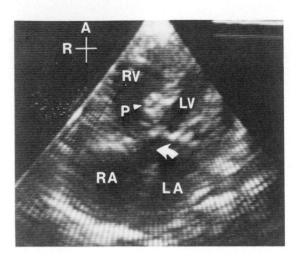

FIG. 5-23. *Apical four-chamber view from a patient with an ostium primum atrial septal defect (arrow) and a tricuspid pouch (P). The absence of echoes in the lower atrial septum adjacent to the atrioventricular valves is the primum atrial septal defect. The echo dropout in the superior portion of the atrial septum is due to either an associated secundum atrial septal defect or the thinness of the fossa ovalis. The right atrium (RA) and right ventricle (RV) are enlarged, and the RV is apex forming. The ventricular septum is intact. A tricuspid pouch is seen protruding into the RV in systole. A, apex; LA, left atrium; LV, left ventricle; R, right.*

The mitral and tricuspid valves are separate and attach by chordae to the crest of the ventricular septum. When the atrioventricular valves close in systole, there is no evidence of a ventricular septal defect. Occasionally, the uppermost portion of the ventricular septum is redundant and protrudes into the right ventricle in systole (Fig. 5-23). These protruberances or tricuspid pouches are commonly associated with ostium primum atrial septal defects.

In the parasternal long-axis view, the mitral valve and left ventricular cavity are abnormally oriented so that the mitral valve opens toward the septum

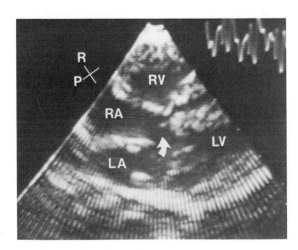

FIG. 5-24. *Subcostal four-chamber view from a patient with an ostium primum atrial septal defect (arrow). The defect is located in the inferior portion of the atrial septum adjacent to the atrioventricular valves. The right atrium (RA) and right ventricle (RV) are enlarged. LA, left atrium; LV, left ventricle; P, posterior; R, right.*

and into the left ventricular outflow tract in diastole. The abnormal mitral valve orientation and attachments give the left ventricular outflow tract an elongated, narrowed appearance in the parasternal long-axis view. This echocardiographic finding is equivalent to the angiographic gooseneck deformity. In addition, the mitral valve is usually thickened and shaggy in appearance and prolapsing.

The cleft anterior mitral valve leaflet can be visualized in the parasternal short-axis view through the left ventricle.[41] Rather than the normal fish-mouth appearance of the mitral valve, the anterior mitral valve leaflet is divided into two portions that separate in diastole (Fig. 5-25).

Ventricular Septal Defect of the Atrioventricular Canal Type. The apical four-chamber view, a posterior plane which passes through the inlet septum, is especially useful for imaging isolated ventricular septal defects of the atrioventricular canal type. When the atrioventricular valves are closed in systole in patients with this defect, no ostium primum atrial septal defect is present (Fig. 5-19). The posterior position of these defects in the area of the inlet septum and the frequent finding of an associated cleft anterior mitral valve leaflet help distinguish ventricular septal defects of the atrioventricular canal type from other types of ventricular septal defect.

Complete Atrioventricular Canal Defect

In complete atrioventricular canal defects, a large central defect involving the lower portion of the atrial septum and the upper portion of the ventricular septum is present. Instead of separate mitral and tricuspid valves, a large common anterior leaflet bridges the atrioventricular canal defect. The morphology and attachments of the common anterior leaflet form the basis for the Rastelli

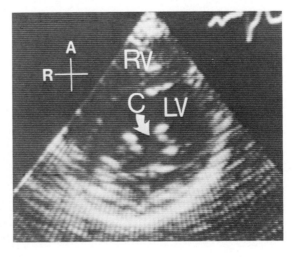

FIG. 5-25. *Parasternal short-axis view at the level of the left ventricle (LV) in a patient with a cleft (C) in the anterior mitral valve leaflet. In diastole, the anterior mitral valve leaflet separates into two portions. A, anterior; R, right; RV, right ventricle.*

classification of complete atrioventricular canal defects.[42] In type A, the common anterior leaflet is divided into separate mitral and tricuspid components with chordal attachments directly to the crest of the ventricular septum. In type B, the common anterior leaflet is divided into separate mitral and tricuspid components with chordal attachments to the right ventricular side of the septum. In type C, an undivided, free-floating common anterior leaflet with no chordal attachments to the ventricular septum is present.

In patients with complete atrioventricular canal defect, the apical and subcostal four-chamber views are most useful for sizing the septal defects and determining the morphology of the common anterior leaflet. When the common anterior leaflet is closed in systole, the full extent of the atrial and ventricular components of the atrioventricular canal defect can be visualized (Fig. 5-26, middle). During diastole in types A and B complete atrioventricular canal defects, the open common anterior leaflet is divided into mitral and tricuspid components (Fig. 5-26, top). In real time, the chordal attachments of the common anterior leaflet to the crest of the ventricular septum in type A and to the right ventricular side of the septum in type B can be seen. During diastole in type C complete atrioventricular canal defect, the common anterior leaflet is undivided and moves across the defect as a straight bar.[40] The bridging common anterior leaflet can also be seen in the parasternal long- and short-axis views (Fig. 5-27).

Abnormalities in the postoperative echocardiogram are common in patients who have undergone surgical repair of a complete atrioventricular canal defect. Cardiac chambers may be enlarged due to residual septal defects or, more commonly, atrioventricular valve insufficiency. Bright echoes can be seen arising from the patch extending from the inferior atrial septum to the uppermost ventricular septum (Fig. 5-26, bottom). The newly created mitral and tricuspid valves are situated at nearly the same level and closer to the cardiac apex than the atrioventricular valves in normal patients (Fig. 5-28). This appearance is related to the abnormal attachments and position of the common anterior leaflet. Residual thickening and prolapse of the new mitral and tricuspid valves is common.

PATENT DUCTUS ARTERIOSUS

Increased pulmonary blood flow and increased pulmonary venous return caused by a left-to-right shunt through a patent ductus arteriosus lead to left atrial and left ventricular enlargement. In premature infants with a patent ductus arteriosus and a compliant left atrium and left ventricle, the left atrial/aortic root ratio measured from the M-mode echocardiogram is useful for assessing indirectly the size of the ductal shunt.[43-46] Because of its ability to image the left atrium in several planes, a more accurate estimate of left atrial size can be obtained from the two-dimensional echocardiogram. Also, in some patients the patent ductus arteriosus can be imaged directly in the parasternal

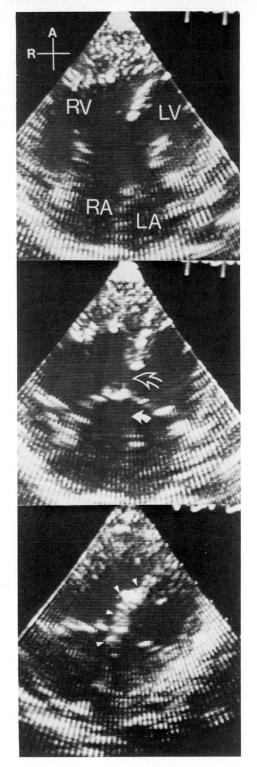

FIG. 5-26. *Apical four-chamber views from a patient with type A complete atrioventricular canal defect.* **Top.** *In diastole, the common anterior leaflet is divided into mitral and tricuspid components. In real time, attachments of these components to the crest of the ventricular septum are seen. A large central defect involving the inferior atrial septum and superior ventricular septum is present. The inferior edge of the atrial septal remnant has a bulbous appearance which gives the atrial septal remnant a matchstick configuration.*[40] *A, apex; LA, left atrium; LV, left ventricle; R, right; RA, right atrium; RV, right ventricle.* **Middle.** *When the common anterior leaflet closes in systole, the sizes of the ventricular (open arrow) and atrial (closed arrow) septal defects can be assessed.* **Bottom.** *Following surgical repair, a highly reflective patch (arrows) can be seen extending from the inferior atrial septum to the upper portion of the ventricular septum.*

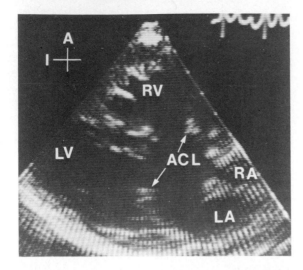

FIG. 5-27. *Parasternal long-axis view oriented toward the tricuspid area in a patient with a type A complete atrioventricular canal defect. A large divided anterior common leaflet (ACL) is seen bridging the septal defect. A, anterior; I, inferior; LA, left atrium; LV, left ventricle; RA, right atrium; RV, right ventricle.*

FIG. 5-28. *Apical four-chamber view from a patient with type A complete atrioventricular canal defect following surgical repair. A highly reflective dacron patch (P) is seen extending over the atrial and ventricular portions of the defect. The newly-created mitral and tricuspid valves are situated at the same level and closer to the cardiac apex than the normal atrioventricular valves. A, apex; LA, left atrium; LV, left ventricle; R, right; RA, right atrium; RV, right ventricle.*

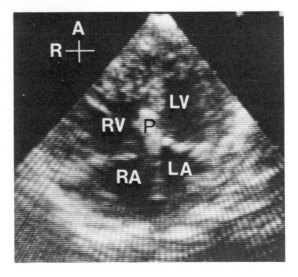

short-axis view.[47] For these reasons, the two-dimensional echocardiogram has become a valuable technique in the noninvasive evaluation of infants with patent ductus arteriosus.

Indirect Evidences of a Patent Ductus Arteriosus

In patients with a large patent ductus arteriosus, the two-dimensional echocardiographic signs of left atrial and left ventricular enlargement are the same as in other defects with left ventricular volume overload. The apical and sub-costal four-chamber views and the parasternal and apical long-axis views are especially useful for detecting enlargement of the left heart and hypercontrac-tility of the left ventricle. In premature and newborn infants with right heart dominance, the atrial septum in the four-chamber views usually bulges toward the left. Prominent reverse bulging of the atrial septum toward the right in the four-chamber views in a premature or newborn infant is strong evidence of left atrial dilatation.

In patent ductus arteriosus with a large diastolic left-to-right shunt, prom-inent pulsations can be seen in the descending aorta in the subcostal long-axis view. Two-dimensional contrast echocardiography using an umbilical artery catheter (see Chap. 4) is another useful technique for proving the existence of a patent ductus arteriosus.

Direct Visualization of the Patent Ductus Arteriosus

The patent ductus arteriosus can sometimes be visualized in the parasternal short-axis view at the base of the heart by angulating the transducer leftward and superiorly through the pulmonary artery bifurcation. In this view, the pat-ent ductus arteriosus is seen arising from the main pulmonary artery between the right and left pulmonary artery branches and connecting to the descend-ing thoracic aorta (Figs. 5-29, 5-30). While it is possible to image a wide, short patent ductus arteriosus in a larger patient, it is extremely difficult to visualize the ductus arteriosus with certainty in the small, premature infant. In order to image a small ductus in the short-axis view, a system with excellent lateral resolution and a high-frequency transducer is necessary. In addition, strict at-tention to gain settings is important because gain settings that are too high can obliterate the patent ductus arteriosus. The patent ductus arteriosus in prema-

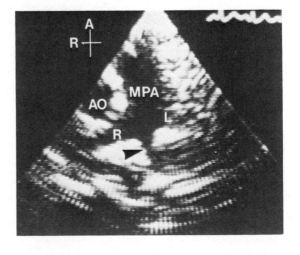

FIG. 5-29. *Parasternal short-axis view through the base of the heart from a patient with a patent ductus arteriosus ((arrow). In order to visualize the patent ductus arteriosus, the transducer is angulated cranially and left-ward toward the pulmonary ar-tery bifurcation. The ductus is seen arising from the main pulmo-nary artery (MPA) between the right (R) and left (L) pulmonary artery branches. A, anterior; AO, aorta; R, right.*

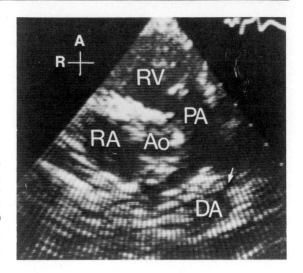

FIG. 5-30. *Parasternal short-axis view through the base of the heart from a patient with a patent ductus arteriosus (arrow). The ductus arteriosus is seen connecting the pulmonary artery (PA) with the descending aorta (DA). A, anterior; Ao, aorta; R, right; RA, right atrium; RV, right ventricle.*

ture infants is often long and tortuous and, even with optimal instrumentation, may not be seen because it passes in and out of the examining plane.

INTRACRANIAL ARTERIOVENOUS MALFORMATION

Intracranial arteriovenous malformation is a rare form of left-to-right shunting. Infants with congestive heart failure and cyanosis caused by this defect are critically ill, and prompt diagnosis is essential. Two-dimensional ultrasonog-

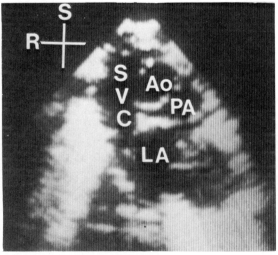

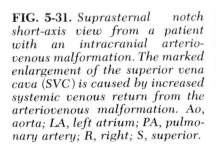

FIG. 5-31. *Suprasternal notch short-axis view from a patient with an intracranial arteriovenous malformation. The marked enlargement of the superior vena cava (SVC) is caused by increased systemic venous return from the arteriovenous malformation. Ao, aorta; LA, left atrium; PA, pulmonary artery; R, right; S, superior.*

raphy provides a rapid, safe, and efficient method for evaluation of the heart and brain in infants with intracranial arteriovenous malformation.

Chamber Size

The large amount of blood flow into the low resistance fistula leads to dilatation of the ascending aorta and carotid arteries that can be detected in the suprasternal notch long-axis view. The increased systemic venous return from the arteriovenous fistula leads to enlargement of the superior vena cava, right atrium, right ventricle, and main pulmonary artery. Dilatation of the superior vena cava and innominate veins can be observed in the suprasternal notch short-axis view (Fig. 5-31). Right atrial, right ventricular, and pulmonary artery enlargement can be seen in the parasternal and subcostal short-axis views and in the apical and subcostal four-chamber views.

Direct Visualization of the Defect

For direct visualization of the intracranial arteriovenous malformation, the transducer is positioned in the anterior fontanel and swept from anterior to posterior in a coronal body plane and from right to left in a sagittal body plane. Also, a transverse view of the brain is obtained by applying the transducer to the temporal bone in a horizontal plane. In all three planes, the arteriovenous malformation appears as a large, fluid-filled structure within the brain (Figs. 4-11, 5-32, 5-33).[48] In some patients, the afferent vessels connecting to the intracranial arteriovenous malformation can be seen (Fig. 5-34).

Definition of Blood Flow Patterns

Shortly after birth when the pulmonary vascular resistances are still elevated, the decrease in total systemic vascular resistance caused by the presence of a large arteriovenous fistula promotes right-to-left ductal shunting. The large venous return to the right atrium from the fistula augments right-to-left atrial shunting. In the presence of the large right-to-left ductal shunt, the pulmonary blood flow and left atrial volume are decreased, and further right-to-left atrial shunting occurs because the flap valve of the foramen ovale remains open.[49] This persistence of fetal circulatory patterns allows microcavitations from a peripheral venous contrast injection to pass from right-to-left at the atrial level, travel in the ascending aorta to the carotid arteries, and opacify the arteriovenous malformation. In this way, the arteriovenous malformation can be separated from other fluid-filled structures (such as the lateral ventricles), which are nonvascular and, therefore, not opacified by contrast echoes (Figs. 4-11, 5-32, 5-33).[48]

Microcavitations reach the fistula, bypass filtration by the systemic capillary bed, and reappear rapidly in the superior vena cava. Superior vena caval recirculation can be detected in the suprasternal notch short-axis view (Fig. 4-13).

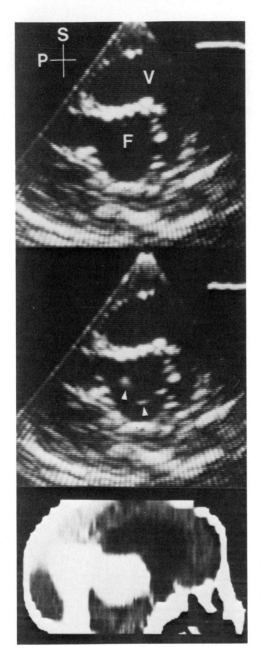

FIG. 5-32. **Top.** *Sagittal view of the brain from a patient with an intracranial arteriovenous malformation. The lateral ventricle (V) is seen as an echo-free space. The echo-free space inferior to the lateral ventricle is a vein of Galen fistula (F). P, posterior; S, superior.* **Middle.** *Following a peripheral venous contrast injection, microcavitations (arrows), which passed from right-to-left at atrial level, are seen in the fistula.* **Bottom.** *Computerized tomography scan in the sagittal plane for comparison. The fistula is opacified by a contrast agent.*

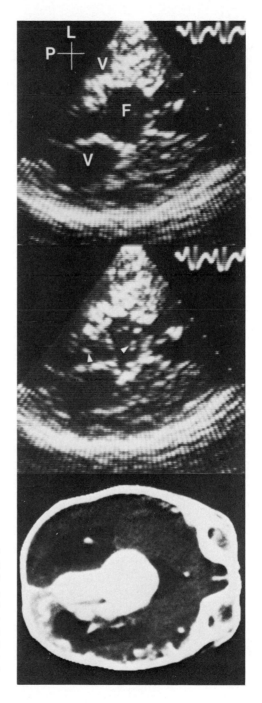

FIG. 5-33. Top. *Transverse view of the brain from a patient with a vein of Galen fistula. The echo-free space between the lateral ventricles (V) is the fistula (F). L, left; P, posterior.* **Middle.** *Following a peripheral venous contrast injection, microcavitations (arrows), which passed from right-to-left at atrial level, are seen in the fistula.* **Bottom.** *Computerized tomography scan with contrast in the transverse plane for comparison.*

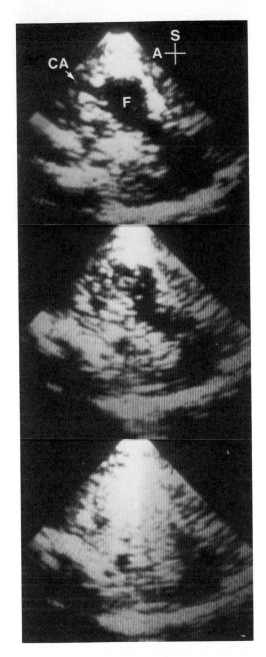

FIG. 5-34. Top. *Sagittal view of the brain from a patient with a vein of Galen fistula (F). An anterior cerebral artery (CA) is seen communicating with the fistula. A, anterior; S, superior.* **Middle.** *Following a peripheral venous contrast injection, microcavitations are seen entering the fistula from the anterior cerebral artery.* **Bottom.** *Most of the fistula is opacified by contrast echoes.*

REFERENCES

1. Diamond MA, Dillon JC, Haine CL, Chang S, Feigenbaum H: Echocardiographic features of atrial septal defect. Circulation 43: 129, 1971
2. Tajik AJ, Gau GT, Ritter DG, Schattenberg TT: Echocardiographic pattern of right ventricular diastolic volume overload in children. Circulation 46: 36, 1972
3. Meyer RA, Schwartz DC, Benzing G III, Kaplan S: Ventricular septum in right ventricular volume overload: An echocardiographic study. Am J Cardiol 30: 349, 1972
4. Kerber RE, Dippel WF, Abboud FM: Abnormal motion of the interventricular septum in right ventricular volume overload. Circulation 48: 86, 1973
5. Hagan AD, Francis GS, Sahn DJ, Karliner JS, Friedman WF, O'Rourke RA: Ultrasound evaluation of systolic anterior septal motion in patients with and without right ventricular volume overload. Circulation 50: 248, 1974
6. Dillon JC, Weyman AE, Feigenbaum H, Eggleton RC, Johnston K: Cross-sectional echocardiographic examination of the interatrial septum. Circulation 55: 115, 1977
7. Lieppe W, Scallion R, Behar VS, Kisslo JA: Two-dimensional echocardiographic findings in atrial septal defect. Circulation 56: 447, 1977
8. Schapira JN, Martin RP, Fowles RE, Popp RL: Single and two dimensional echocardiographic features of the interatrial septum in normal subjects and patients with an atrial septal defect. Am J Cardiol 43: 816, 1979
9. Bierman FZ, Williams RG: Subxiphoid two-dimensional imaging of the interatrial septum in infants and neonates with congenital heart disease. Circulation 60: 80, 1979
10. Tajik AJ, Seward JB, Giuliani ER: Ventricular septal motion: Clinical echocardiographic correlations. Cardiovasc Clin 9: 209, 1978
11. Weyman AE, Wann S, Feigenbaum H, Dillon JC: Mechanism of abnormal septal motion in patients with right ventricular volume overload: A cross-sectional echocardiographic study. Circulation 54: 179, 1976
12. Rosenquist GC, Sweeny LJ, Ruckman RN, McAllister HA: Atrial septal thickness and area in normal heart specimens and in those with ostium secundum atrial septal defects. J Clin Ultrasound 7: 345, 1979
13. Goor DA, Lillehei CW: Congenital Malformations of the Heart. New York, Grune and Stratton, 1975, pp 1–37
14. Anderson RH: Embryology of the ventricular septum. In: Paediatric Cardiology. RH Anderson, EA Shinebourne, eds. London, Churchill Livingstone, 1978, pp 103–112
15. King DL, Steeg CN, Ellis K: Visualization of ventricular septal defects by cardiac ultrasonography. Circulation 48: 1215, 1973
16. Seward JB, Tajik AJ, Hagler DJ, Mair DD: Visualization of isolated ventricular septal defect with wide-angle two-dimensional sector echocardiography. Circulation 58 (Suppl II): II-202, 1978
17. Cheatham JP, Latson LA, Gutgesell HP: Ventricular septal defect in infancy: Detection by two-dimensional echocardiography. Circulation 60 (Suppl II): II-60, 1979
18. Canale JM, Sahn DJ, Allen HD, Goldberg SJ: Factors affecting real-time cross-sectional echocardiographic imaging of ventricular septal defects. Am J Cardiol 45: 457, 1980

19. Van Mill GJ: The echocardiography of ventricular septal defects. In: Echocardiography. Hunter S (ed.) London, Churchill Livingstone, 1981

20. Bierman FZ, Fellows K, Williams RG: Prospective identification of ventricular septal defects in infancy using subxiphoid two-dimensional echocardiography. Circulation 62: 807, 1980

21. Draelos ZK, Goldberg SJ, Sahn DJ: How accurate is the ultrasonically imaged size of a ventricular septal defect (VSD)? Circulation 62 (Suppl III): III-164, 1980

22. Bloom KR, Rodriques L, Swan EM: Echocardiographic evaluation of left-to-right shunt in ventricular septal defect and persistent ductus arteriosus. Br Heart J 39: 260, 1977

23. Sahn DJ, Vaucher Y, Williams DE, Allen HD, Goldberg SJ, Friedman WF: Echocardiographic detection of large left-to-right shunts and cardiomyopathies in infants and children. Am J Cardiol 38: 73, 1976

24. Lester LA, Vitullo D, Sodt P, Hutcheon N, Arcilla R: An evaluation of the left atrial/aortic root ratio in children with ventricular septal defect. Circulation 60: 364, 1979

25. Freedom RM, White RD, Pieroni DR, Varghese PJ, Krovetz LJ, Rowe RD: The natural history of the so-called aneurysm of the membranous ventricular septum in childhood. Circulation 49: 375, 1974

26. Hoffman JIE, Rudolph AM: The natural history of ventricular septal defects in infancy. Am J Cardiol 16: 634, 1965

27. Nugent EW, Freedom RM, Rowe RD, Wagner HR, Rees JK: Aneurysm of the membranous septum in ventricular septal defect. Circulation 56 (Suppl I): I-82, 1977

28. Sahn DJ, Kirkpatrick SE, Friedman WF: Echocardiographic recognition of ventricular septal aneurysm: A case report. J Clin Ultrasound 3: 297, 1975

29. Snider AR, Silverman NH, Schiller NB, Ports TA: Echocardiographic evaluation of ventricular septal aneurysms. Circulation 59: 920, 1979

30. Williams RG, Rudd M: Echocardiographic features of endocardial cushion defects. Circulation 49: 418, 1974

31. Pieroni DR, Homcy E, Freedom RM: Echocardiography in atrioventricular canal defect: A clinical spectrum. Am J Cardiol 35: 54, 1975

32. Eshaghpour E, Turnoff HB, Kingsley B, Kawai N, Linhart JW: Echocardiography in endocardial cushion defects: A preoperative and postoperative study. Chest 68: 172, 1975

33. Komatsu Y, Nagai Y, Shibuya M, Takao A, Hirosawa K: Echocardiographic analysis of intracardiac anatomy in endocardial cushion defect. Am Heart J 91: 210, 1976

34. Bass JL, Bessinger FB Jr, Lawrence C: Echocardiographic differentiation of partial and complete atrioventricular canal. Circulation 57: 1144, 1978

35. Bloom KR, Freedom RM, Williams CM, Trusler GA, Rowe RD: Echocardiographic recognition of atrioventricular valve stenosis associated with endocardial cushion defect: Pathologic and surgical correlates. Am J Cardiol 44: 1326, 1979

36. Mehta S, Hirschfeld S, Riggs T, Liebman J: Echocardiographic estimation of ventricular hypoplasia in complete atrioventricular canal. Circulation 59: 888, 1979

37. Sahn DJ, Terry RW, O'Rourke R, Leopold G, Friedman WF: Multiple crystal echocardiographic evaluation of endocardial cushion defect. Circulation 50: 25, 1974

38. Yoshikawa J, Owaki T, Kato H, Tomita Y, Baba K, Tanaka K: Echocardiographic diagnosis of endocardial cushion defects. Jap Heart J 16: 1, 1975

39. Beppu S, Nimura Y, Nagata S, Tamai M, Matsuo H, Matsumoto M, Kawashima Y,

Sakakibara H, Abe H: Diagnosis of endocardial cushion defect with cross-sectional and M-mode scanning echocardiography: Differentiation from secundum atrial septal defect. Br Heart J 38: 911, 1976

40. Hagler DJ, Tajik AJ, Seward JB, Mair DD, Ritter DG: Real-time wide-angle sector echocardiography: Atrioventricular canal defects. Circulation 59: 140, 1979

41. Beppu S, Nimura Y, Sakakibara H, Nagata S, Park Y-D, Baba K, Naito Y, Ohta M, Kamiya T, Koyanagi H, Fujita T: Mitral cleft in ostium primum atrial septal defect assessed by cross-sectional echocardiography. Circulation 62: 1099, 1980

42. Rastelli GC, Kirklin JW, Titus JL: Anatomic observations on complete form of persistent common atrioventricular canal with special reference to atrioventricular valves. Mayo Clin Proc 41: 296, 1966

43. Silverman NH, Lewis AB, Heymann MA, Rudolph AM: Echocardiographic assessment of ductus arteriosus shunt in premature infants. Circulation 50: 821, 1974

44. Laird WP, Fixler DE: Echocardiography of premature infants with pulmonary disease: A noninvasive method for detecting large ductal left-to-right shunts. Radiology 122: 455, 1977

45. Baylen B, Meyer RA, Korfhagen J, Benzing G III, Bubb ME, Kaplan S: Left ventricular performance in the critically ill premature infant with patent ductus arteriosus and pulmonary disease. Circulation 55: 182, 1977

46. Goldberg SJ, Allen HD, Sahn DJ: Echocardiographic detection and management of patent ductus arteriosus and neonates with respiratory distress syndrome: A two-and-one-half year prospective study. J Clin Ultrasound 5: 161, 1977

47. Sahn DJ, Allen HD: Real-time cross-sectional echocardiographic imaging and measurement of the patent ductus arteriosus in infants and children. Circulation 58: 343, 1978

48. Snider AR, Soifer SJ, Silverman NH: Detection of intracranial arteriovenous fistula by two-dimensional ultrasonography. Circulation 63: 1179, 1981

49. Cumming GR: Circulation in neonates with intracranial arteriovenous fistula and cardiac failure. Am J Cardiol 45: 1019, 1980

CHAPTER 6

Ventricular Outflow Obstruction

Ventricular outflow obstruction caused by a fixed anatomic lesion can occur in the valvar, subvalvar, or supravalvar region of the outflow tract. Two-dimensional echocardiography is a valuable technique for determining the anatomic location and type of obstructing lesion and for detecting frequently associated defects.

AORTIC VALVE STENOSIS

In real time, the normal aortic valve cusps are thin structures with brisk, unrestricted mobility. In patients with aortic valve stenosis, the aortic valve cusps are thickened and domed (Fig. 6-1). In real time, the stiffly-moving cusps are restricted in lateral mobility[1] and exhibit diminished cusp separation.[2,3] The parasternal and apical long-axis views and the parasternal and subcostal short-axis views are especially useful for evaluating the stenotic aortic valve.

Patients with moderate-to-severe aortic valve stenosis usually have concentric hypertrophy of the left ventricle on the two-dimensional echocardiogram (Fig. 6-2). The aortic valve annulus may be narrowed (Fig. 6-2), and there is usually evidence of poststenotic dilatation of the ascending aorta in the long axis and suprasternal notch views.

Anatomic Type

Aortic valve stenosis can occur with a tricuspid, bicuspid, or unicuspid aortic valve. In the closed position, the parasternal short-axis view shows the com-

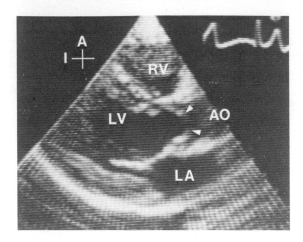

FIG. 6-1. *Parasternal long-axis view from a patient with aortic valve stenosis. The aortic valve cusps (arrows) are thickened and domed, and there is diminished cusp separation. A, anterior; AO, aorta; I, inferior; LA, left atrium; LV, left ventricle; RV, right ventricle.*

missures of the normal tricuspid aortic valve forming a Y or inverted Mercedes-Benz sign. Because of the rapid movement of the normally thin aortic valve leaflets and the movement of the aortic valve annulus in and out of the examining plane, it is not always possible to demonstrate the entire Y pattern in some normal patients.[4] In patients with aortic valve stenosis and a tricuspid aortic valve, the thickening of the edges of the aortic leaflets makes visualization of the Y pattern easier (Figs. 6-3, 6-4). Stenotic tricuspid aortic valves can open centrally (Fig. 6-3) or eccentrically due to partial fusion of commissures (Fig. 6-4).

In the stenotic bicuspid aortic valve, the thickened edges of the two cusps form a single diastolic closure line, which may be centrally (Fig. 6-5) or eccentrically (Fig. 6-6) located in the aortic root.[5] In the parasternal short-axis view, the diastolic closure line of a bicuspid aortic valve can be oriented in a vertical or horizontal direction. In patients with a bicuspid aortic valve that is not yet thickened and stenotic, the diastolic closure line is not so prominent and differentiation from a normal tricuspid valve with incomplete visualization of the Y pattern may be difficult. Also, echoes reflected from a raphe or fused commissural ridge can make a bicuspid aortic valve appear to be tricuspid. In order to minimize errors when determining the number of cusps, the aortic valve should be examined from multiple angles and locations, and the videotape should be carefully reviewed in slow motion.

In a high percentage of bicuspid aortic valves, we have seen a reverse doming of the valve into the left ventricular outflow tract in diastole (Fig. 6-7). The reverse doming involves the entire aortic valve and is quite different in appearance from prolapse of an aortic valve cusp seen in patients with supracristal ventricular septal defects or rheumatic aortic insufficiency (see Chapter 8). The etiology and significance of reverse doming remains to be determined.

Unicuspid aortic valves are commonly found in infants with critical aortic stenosis. On the two-dimensional echocardiogram, these valves are extremely

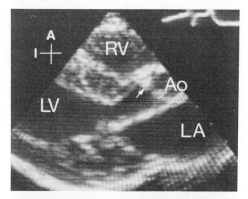

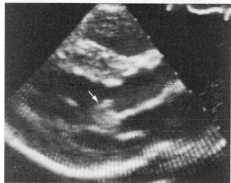

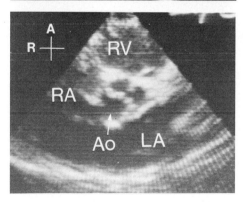

FIG. 6-2. *Two-dimensional echocardiogram from a 16-year-old male who had undergone aortic valvotomy at age 3 for a severely stenotic bicuspid valve.* **Top.** *The parasternal long-axis view in diastole shows evidence of severe residual aortic valve stenosis. There is concentric hypertrophy of the left ventricle (LV). The aortic valve (arrow) is thickened and the aortic annulus is small. A, anterior; Ao, aorta; I, inferior; LA, left atrium; RV, right ventricle.* **Middle.** *In systole, the myocardial hypertrophy creates a dynamic subaortic stenosis causing systolic anterior motion of the mitral valve (arrow).* **Bottom.** *Parasternal short-axis view through the base of the heart. The aortic valve appears to be tricuspid because of the surgically opened raphe. Note the thickened margins of the valve leaflets and the small aortic annulus. R, right; RA, right atrium.*

thickened and dysplastic. In systole, a severely domed aortic valve with a small orifice is seen (Fig. 6-8).[4] The aortic valve annulus and ascending aorta are often narrowed. Shortly after birth, the left ventricle is usually thin walled and poorly contractile. In time hypertrophy develops, and the left ventricle may appear concentrically thickened and contracted. Often bright echoes can be seen arising from the endocardium in areas where there is diffuse endocardial fibroelastosis. Because of the thickness of the aortic valve and the narrowness of the aortic annulus, this defect may be difficult to distinguish from the

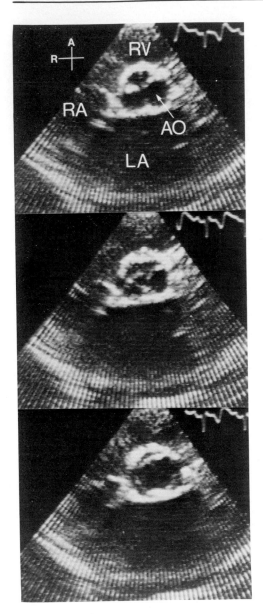

FIG. 6-3. **Top.** *Parasternal short-axis view in diastole from a patient with a stenotic tricuspid aortic valve. The thickened edges of the closed aortic valve cusps create a Y pattern. A, anterior; AO, aorta; LA, left atrium; R, right; RA, right atrium; RV, right ventricle.* **Middle and Bottom.** *In systole, the aortic valve orifice is outlined by the thickened margins of the valve leaflets. The aortic orifice is centrally located in the aortic root.*

hypoplastic left heart syndrome. We believe that any infant with a left ventricular cavity and either an aortic valve annulus greater than 5 mm[4] or evidence of a patent aortic valve should be considered to have critical aortic stenosis until proved otherwise. Aortic valve patency can be determined by direct visualization in some cases or by contrast echocardiography in other cases (see Chapter 11).

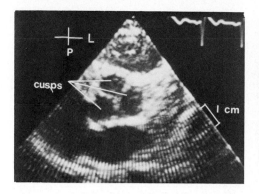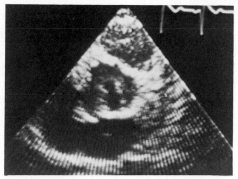

FIG. 6-4. Left. *Parasternal short-axis view in diastole from a patient with a stenotic tricuspid aortic valve. The thickened edges of the valve cusps form a Y pattern. L, left; P, posterior.* **Right.** *In systole, the aortic valve opens eccentrically because of partial fusion of the commissures.*

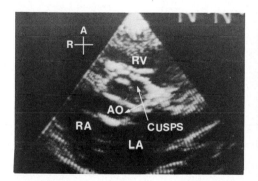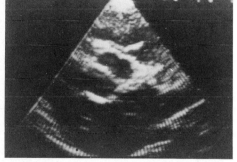

FIG. 6-5. *Parasternal short-axis views from a patient with a stenotic bicuspid aortic valve.* **Left.** *In systole the aortic orifice and the two aortic cusps can be seen. A, anterior; AO, aorta; LA, left atrium; R, right; RA, right atrium; RV, right ventricle.* **Right.** *In diastole a single diastolic closure line is centrally located in the aortic root.*

Estimation of Severity of Aortic Stenosis

Using Laplace's Law for calculating wall tension, several investigators have derived formulas for estimating the severity of the aortic stenosis from the M-mode echocardiogram.[6-12] The echocardiographic measurements required in these formulas are not easily derived from the two-dimensional display; therefore, other means of estimating the severity of aortic stenosis from the two-dimensional echocardiogram were sought. Weyman and colleagues[3] have used the ratio of the maximum cusp separation to the aortic root diameter to estimate the severity of the stenosis; however, errors in the ratio can occur

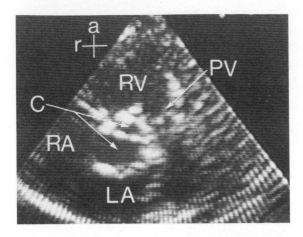

FIG. 6-6. *Parasternal short-axis view from a patient with a stenotic bicuspid aortic valve. The single diastolic closure line is eccentrically positioned in the aortic root and the two aortic valve cusps (C) are unequal in size. a, anterior; LA, left atrium; PV, pulmonary valve; r, right; RA, right atrium; RV, right ventricle.*

FIG. 6-7. *Parasternal long-axis view from a patient with a bicuspid aortic valve. There is reverse doming of the aortic valve (arrows) into the left ventricular outflow tract in diastole. A, anterior; AO, aorta; I, inferior; LA, left atrium; LV, left ventricle; RV, right ventricle.*

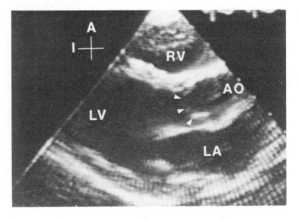

because of beam angulation or improper gain settings.[13] Two-dimensional echocardiographic findings such as cusp separation, doming, and poststenotic dilatation provide an accurate qualitative assessment of the severity of aortic stenosis, but we continue to rely on the Laplace relationships and serial measurements of the left ventricular posterior wall thickness from the M-mode echocardiogram to predict the severity of the stenosis.

SUBVALVAR AORTIC STENOSIS

Several M-mode echocardiographic findings including early closure of the aortic valve, coarse systolic aortic valve flutter, and a diminished mitral-to-septal distance in the left ventricular outflow tract have been described in pa-

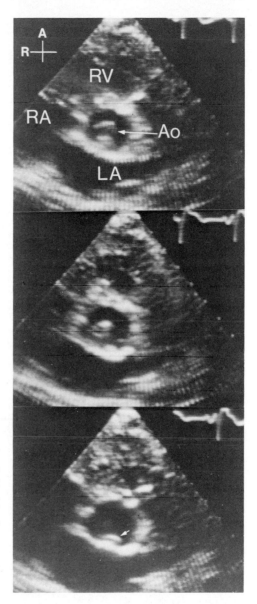

FIG. 6-8. *Parasternal short-axis views from a patient with a stenotic, unicuspid aortic valve.* **Top.** *At the time of maximum systolic excursion the valve opening is severely restricted. A, anterior; Ao, aorta; LA, left atrium; R, right; RA, right atrium; RV, right ventricle.* **Top and Middle.** *The valve has a central orifice with no distinct cusps.* **Bottom.** *In diastole, the valve closure (arrow) is eccentric and located adjacent to the posterior aortic root.*

tients with subvalvar aortic stenosis.[14,15] Early closure of the aortic valve is invariably present in patients with subaortic stenosis but is not specific for this defect. Although direct recording of a membrane in the left ventricular outflow tract has been possible, in most instances the M-mode echocardiogram does not indicate the exact anatomy of the subaortic stenosis. The anatomic type of subaortic stenosis can be determined from the two-dimensional echocardiogram[1,16,17]; however, we continue to use the Laplace formulas and the left ventricular posterior wall thickness measured from the M-mode echocardiogram to predict the severity of the obstruction.

The anatomic types of congenital subaortic stenosis include discrete subvalvar membrane, fibromuscular collar, and tunnel subaortic stenosis. The discrete fibrous membrane is best seen in the parasternal and apical long-axis views as a thin echo stretching across the left ventricular outflow tract just beneath the aortic valve (Figs. 6-9 and 6-10). The overall cardiac motion can make visualization of the thin membrane difficult, and in most cases, the membrane cannot be seen in its entirety. Careful attention to gain and reject settings is necessary for optimal imaging of the membrane. In most patients

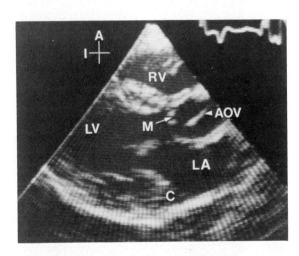

FIG. 6-9. *Parasternal long-axis view from a patient with subaortic stenosis caused by a discrete fibrous membrane (M). The membrane is positioned in the left ventricular outflow tract just beneath the aortic valve (AOV). A, anterior; C, coronary sinus; I, inferior; LA, left atrium; LV, left ventricle; RV, right ventricle.*

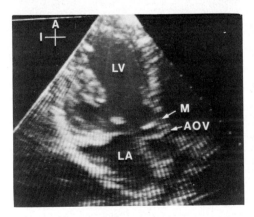 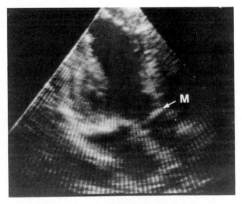

FIG. 6-10. *Apical long-axis views in diastole* (**left**) *and systole* (**right**) *from a patient with a discrete subaortic membrane (M). The membrane stretches across the left ventricular outflow just beneath the aortic valve (AOV). A, anterior; I, inferior; LA, left atrium; LV, left ventricle.*

with a thin subaortic membrane, surgical resection of the membrane can be performed completely and relatively easily. In a few patients, the subaortic membrane is large and redundant and inserts into the midportion of the anterior leaflet of the mitral valve (Fig. 6-11). Surgical resection in these patients carries the risk of damage to the mitral valve leaflets.

The fibromuscular collar is a form of subaortic stenosis involving a more extensive area of the left ventricular outflow tract and is, therefore, less amenable to surgical resection. In the parasternal and apical long-axis views of this defect, a thick fibrous shelf projects anteriorly and posteriorly into the outflow tract (Fig. 6-12). Tunnel subaortic stenosis represents the most extensive form of fibromuscular subaortic stenosis.

Patients with subaortic stenosis frequently have a thickened aortic valve and/or evidence of aortic insufficiency on the two-dimensional echocardiogram. These findings may be due to an associated congenital aortic valve stenosis or damage to a previously normal aortic valve by the subaortic jet.

SUPRAVALVAR AORTIC STENOSIS

In supravalvar aortic stenosis, an area of narrowing (which can be localized or extensive) is present above the coronary arteries at the superior border of the sinuses of Valsalva. In the parasternal and apical long-axis views, the supravalvar aortic constriction can vary in severity and location from a discrete membrane to hypoplasia of the entire ascending aorta. In most instances, there is an hourglass deformity of the external aspects of the aorta with a corresponding narrowing of the aortic lumen (Fig. 6-13).[1,18]

Two-dimensional echocardiography may underestimate the severity of the supravalvar aortic stenosis by failing to image the full extent of the endocardial obstruction.[4] In addition, artifactual narrowing of the ascending aorta

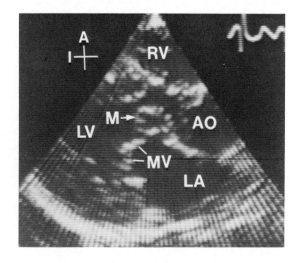

FIG. 6-11. *Parasternal long-axis view from a patient with subaortic stenosis due to a discrete fibrous membrane (M). The membrane is large and redundant and inserts into the midportion of the anterior mitral valve (MV) leaflet. There is concentric hypertrophy of the left ventricle (LV). A, anterior; AO, aorta; I, inferior; LA, left atrium; RV, right ventricle.*

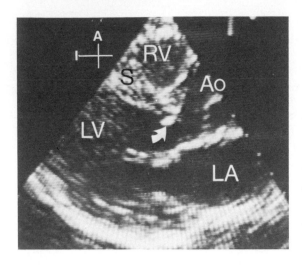

FIG. 6-12. *Parasternal long-axis view from a patient with subaortic stenosis due to a fibromuscular collar (arrow). A thickened, fibromuscular shelf is seen projecting into the left ventricular outflow tract. A, anterior; Ao, aorta; I, inferior; LA, left atrium; LV, left ventricle; RV, right ventricle; S, septum.*

caused by lateral resolution errors can mimic the hourglass deformity. False positive diagnoses can also occur in patients with dilated sinuses of Valsalva. When supravalvar aortic stenosis is detected on the two-dimensional echocardiogram, a search should be made for commonly associated defects such as peripheral pulmonic stenosis.

COARCTATION AND INTERRUPTION OF THE AORTA

Chamber Size

In the perinatal period, infants with coarctation or interruption of the aorta usually have a poorly contractile left ventricle of normal thickness. The aortic obstruction and noncompliant left ventricle lead to left atrial hypertension and dilatation. In the four-chamber views, the left atrium and pulmonary

FIG. 6-13. *Parasternal long-axis view from a patient with supravalvar aortic stenosis. An hourglass type of constriction is seen on the external aspects of the aorta (arrows) with a corresponding narrowing of the aortic lumen. A, anterior; AO, aorta; I, inferior; LA, left atrium; LV, left ventricle; RV, right ventricle.*

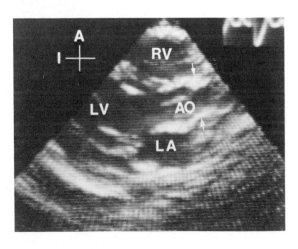

veins are dilated, and the atrial septum bulges prominently toward the right. Also, the right atrium, right ventricle, and main pulmonary artery are dilated. The right ventricle is usually thickened and apex forming in the four-chamber views. In the parasternal and subcostal short-axis views, bright echoes arise from the pulmonary valve suggesting pulmonary artery hypertension.

Following medical intervention or the passage of time in patients with coarctation, the left ventricular function usually returns to normal and the left ventricle thickens. Signs of right heart enlargement can persist for several months.[19]

Direct Visualization of the Defect

In the suprasternal notch long-axis view, the coarctation of the aorta is seen as an area of narrowing in the descending thoracic aorta just beyond the origin of the left subclavian artery (Fig. 6-14).[20,21] Distal to the area of narrowing, there is poststenotic dilatation of the descending aorta. Usually, pominent pulsations are seen in the ascending aorta; however, pulsations in the descending aorta in the suprasternal notch and subcostal views are markedly diminished.

Limitations in lateral resolution can make the normal descending aorta appear narrowed in the suprasternal notch long-axis view and can lead to a false positive diagnosis of coarctation. To avoid this misinterpretation, poststenotic dilatation of the descending aorta and diminished descending aorta pulsations should be noted before making the diagnosis of coarctation. In patients with aortic coarctation, associated lesions such as bicuspid aortic valve, ventricular septal defect, subaortic stenosis, and supravalvar mitral ring should be sought.

In patients who have undergone surgical repair of the coarctation using synthetic material, the bright echoes arising from the patch or graft can create the appearance of residual aortic narrowing (Fig. 6-15). In these patients, the descending aorta pulsation is probably a better indicator of the adequacy of the repair.

In the suprasternal notch long-axis view, interruption of the aorta is seen as an area of atresia or discontinuity in the aortic arch (Fig. 6-16). The area of discontinuity can occur either between the right and left common carotid arteries, between the left common carotid and left subclavian arteries, or beyond the origin of the left subclavian artery. In each type of interruption, the right subclavian artery can arise normally or aberrantly distal to the left subclavian artery. In some patients, the origin of the vessels to the head and neck can be seen clearly. Usually, the ascending aorta is reduced in size and there is an associated ventricular septal defect or aortopulmonary window.

SYSTEMIC HYPERTENSION

Patients with long-standing, severe systemic hypertension can develop concentric left ventricular hypertrophy.[22] On the two-dimensional echocardio-

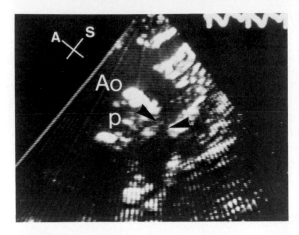

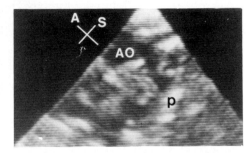

FIG. 6-14. *Suprasternal notch long-axis view from a patient with coarctation of the aorta. An area of narrowing is seen just beyond the origin of the left subclavian artery (arrows). There is poststenotic dilatation of the descending aorta. A, anterior; Ao, aorta; p, right pulmonary artery; S, superior.*

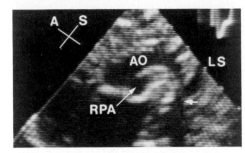

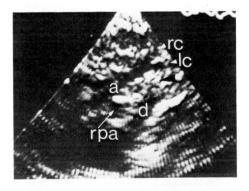

FIG. 6-15. **Left.** *Suprasternal notch long-axis view from an infant with a coarctation (arrow) of the aorta (AO) just beyond the origin of the left subclavian artery (LS). There is poststenotic dilatation of the descending aorta. A, anterior; RPA, right pulmonary artery; S, superior.* **Right.** *Suprasternal notch long-axis view from the same patient following patch (P) repair of the coarctation. The bright echoes arising from the patch cause the aorta (AO) to appear narrowed. A, anterior; S, superior.*

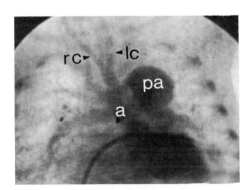

FIG. 6-16. **Left.** *Frame from an anteroposterior cineangiogram in a newborn infant with interruption of the aorta. The right common carotid (rc) and left common carotid (lc) arteries arose from the ascending aorta (a) proximal to the interruption. Both subclavian arteries arose from the descending aorta. pa, main pulmonary artery.* **Right.** *Suprasternal notch long-axis view from the same infant showing the right and left common carotid arteries (rc and lc) arising from the ascending aorta (a) proximal to the interruption (black arrow). The subclavian arteries cannot be seen in this frame. d, descending aorta; rpa, right pulmonary artery.*

gram, the left ventricle is uniformly thickened (Figs. 6-17 and 6-18). In the parasternal short-axis view, the left coronary artery and its branches are usually enlarged because of increased coronary blood flow to the increased left ventricular mass (Fig. 6-19). When the two-dimensional echocardiogram shows signs of left ventricular hypertrophy, a careful search for fixed anatomic defects causing left ventricular outflow tract obstruction should be made. In the late stages of systemic hypertension, the left atrium and left ventricle dilate and left ventricular contractility decreases.

PULMONARY VALVE STENOSIS

In the parasternal and subcostal short-axis views of the normal patient, the pulmonary valve leaflets are thin structures with rapid, unrestricted movement. In patients with pulmonary valve stenosis, the valve leaflets are thickened and have restricted lateral mobility.[23] The valve can vary from a dysplastic, domed, poorly formed valve (Fig. 6-20) to a well-formed, slightly thickened, tricuspid pulmonic valve (Fig. 6-21). The pulmonary valve annulus can vary from extremely small (Fig. 6-20) to normal (Fig. 6-21). Frequently, only a pinhole opening is present at the tip of the domed pulmonic valve in systole. In the neonatal period, the echocardiographic diagnosis of pulmonary stenosis should not be made on the basis of pulmonary valve thickening alone as pulmonary artery hypertension in the newborn period can also lead to a thickened pulmonary valve on the two-dimensional echocardiogram.

The jet stream passing through the stenotic pulmonic valve causes poststenotic dilatation of the main pulmonary artery that can be seen in the parasternal short-axis view and the suprasternal notch views. In these planes, the main pulmonary artery is markedly enlarged; however, the distal right and left pulmonary artery branches are normal in size (Figs. 6-20 and 6-22).

Although the appearance of the pulmonary valve and the valve annulus on the two-dimensional echocardiogram provide a qualitative assessment of the severity of the pulmonic stenosis, we still rely on the right ventricular anterior wall thickness measured from the M-mode echocardiogram to assess the amount of obstruction. In the apical and subcostal four-chamber views, the thickened right ventricle is often apex forming and has a prominent moderator band and septoparietal trabeculations. In severe pulmonic stenosis with a noncompliant right ventricle, signs of right atrial hypertension can be seen in the four-chamber views. The right atrium is enlarged and the atrial septum bulges prominently toward the left. During contrast echocardiography in severe pulmonic stenosis, a right-to-left shunt through the foramen ovale is frequently seen. The thickening of the right ventricle and pulmonary valve normally seen in the perinatal period can be difficult to distinguish from pulmonary stenosis with a normal sized pulmonary annulus.

In patients who have undergone pulmonary valvotomy, hypertrophy of the right ventricle on the two-dimensional echocardiogram can indicate failure of regression of thickened right ventricular muscle rather than significant

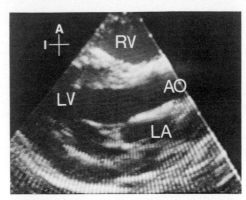

FIG. 6-17. **Top.** *Parasternal long-axis view from a patient with long-standing systemic hypertension caused by renal disease. There is concentric thickening of the left ventricle (LV) and no evidence of subvalvar or valvar aortic stenosis. A, anterior, AO, aorta; I, inferior; LA, left atrium; RV, right ventricle.* **Bottom.** *Subcostal four-chamber view from the same patient showing marked thickening of the septum (S) and left ventricular wall (LVW). I, inferior; LA, left atrium; LV, left ventricle; R, right; RA, right atrium; RV, right ventricle.*

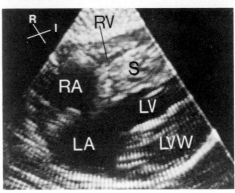

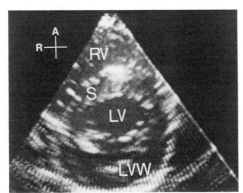

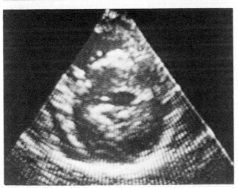

FIG. 6-18. *Parasternal short-axis views through the left ventricle (LV) from the same patient as in Figure 6-17.* **Top.** *the septum (S) and left ventricular wall (LVW) are concentrically thickened. In systole (***bottom***), the left ventricular cavity is nearly obliterated. A, anterior; R, right; RV, right ventricle.*

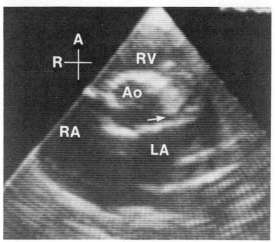

FIG. 6-19. *Parasternal short-axis view through the base of the heart in the same patient as in Figures 6-17 and 6-18. The left main coronary artery (arrow) and its two branches are enlarged because of increased coronary blood flow to the increased left ventricular mass. A, anterior; Ao, aorta; LA, left atrium; R, right; RA, right atrium; RV, right ventricle.*

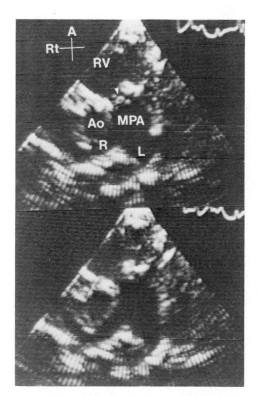

FIG. 6-20. *Parasternal short-axis views through the base of the heart in diastole (**top**) and systole (**bottom**) from a patient with severe pulmonary valve stenosis. The pulmonary valve (arrow) is thickened and the annulus is severely narrowed. There is poststenotic dilatation of the main pulmonary artery (MPA). A, anterior; Ao, aorta; L, left pulmonary artery; R, right pulmonary artery; Rt, right; RV, right ventricle.*

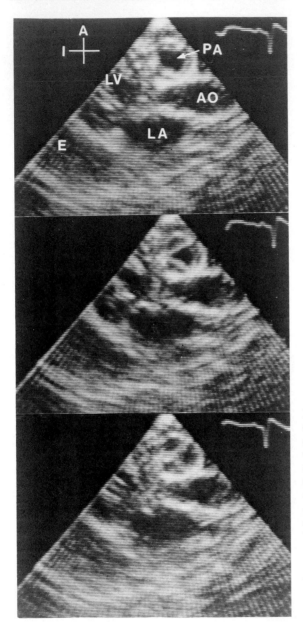

FIG. 6-21. *Parasternal long-axis views from a patient who had recently undergone pulmonary val-votomy. Because of an unusual orientation of the right ventricular outflow tract, the pulmonary artery (PA) can be seen in cross section in the parasternal long-axis view. The thickened edges of the three pulmonary valve cusps are clearly seen. Note that the pulmonary annulus is normal sized. A posterior pericardial effusion (E) is present. A, anterior; AO, aorta; I, inferior; LA, left atrium; LV, left ventricle.*

residual pulmonic stenosis. After pulmonary valvotomy, most patients show evidence of pulmonary insufficiency on the two-dimensional echocardiogram. Right ventricular enlargement, paradoxical septal motion, and vigorous right ventricular ejection can be seen in the four-chamber and short-axis views. With significant pulmonary insufficiency and a low pulmonary artery diastolic pressure, prominent pulsation of the right pulmonary artery can be visualized in the suprasternal notch long-axis view.

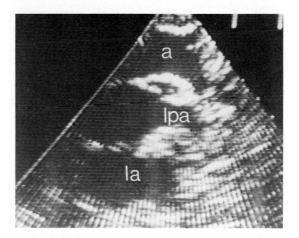

FIG. 6-22. *Suprasternal notch long-axis view from a patient with pulmonary valve stenosis. There is marked poststenotic dilatation of the main pulmonary artery. The left pulmonary artery (lpa) is of normal size. a, aorta; la, left atrium.*

REFERENCES

1. Williams DE, Sahn DJ, Friedman WF: Cross-sectional echocardiographic localization of sites of left ventricular outflow tract obstruction. Am J Cardiol 37: 250, 1976
2. Chang S, Clements S, Chang J: Aortic stenosis: Echocardiographic cusp separation and surgical description of aortic valve in 22 patients. Am J Cardiol 39: 499, 1977
3. Weyman AE, Feigenbaum H, Hurwitz RA, Girod DA, Dillon JC: Cross-sectional echocardiographic assessment of the severity of aortic stenosis in children. Circulation 55: 773, 1977
4. Goldberg SJ, Allen HD, Sahn DJ: Pediatric and Adolescent Echocardiography: A Handbook. Chicago, Year Book Medical Publishers, 1980
5. Fowles RE, Martin RP, Abrams JM, Schapira JN, French JW, Popp RL: Two-dimensional echocardiographic features of bicuspid aortic valve. Chest 75: 434, 1979
6. Bennett DH, Evans DW, Raj MVJ: Echocardiographic left ventricular dimensions in pressure and volume overload: Their use in assessing aortic stenosis. Br Heart J 37: 971, 1975
7. Glanz S, Hellenbrand WE, Berman MA, Talner NH: Echocardiographic assessment of the severity of aortic stenosis in children and adolescents. Am J Cardiol 38: 620, 1976
8. Aziz KU, van Grondelle A, Paul MH, Muster AJ: Echocardiographic assessment of the relation between left ventricular wall and cavity dimension and peak systolic pressure in children with aortic stenosis. Am J Cardiol 40: 775, 1977
9. Johnson GL, Meyer RA, Schwartz DC, Korfhagen J, Kaplan S: Echocardiographic evaluation of fixed left ventricular outlet obstruction in children: Pre- and postoperative assessment of ventricular systolic pressures. Circulation 56: 299, 1977
10. Blackwood RA, Bloom KR, Williams CM: Aortic stenosis in children: Experience with echocardiographic prediction of severity. Circulation 57: 263, 1978
11. Gewitz MH, Werner JC, Kleinman CS, Hellenbrand WE, Talner NS, Taunt KA: Role of echocardiography in aortic stenosis: Pre- and postoperative studies. Am J Cardiol 43: 67, 1979
12. Bass JL, Einzig S, Hong CY, Moller JH: Echocardiographic screening to assess the severity of congenital aortic valve stenosis in children. Am J Cardiol 44: 82, 1979

13. DeMaria AN, Bommer W, Joye J, Lee G, Bouteller J, Mason DT: Value and limitations of cross-sectional echocardiography of the aortic valve in the diagnosis and quantification of valvular aortic stenosis. Circulation 62: 304, 1980

14. Popp RL, Silverman JF, French JW, Stinson EB, Harrison DC: Echocardiographic findings in discrete subvalvular aortic stenosis. Circulation 49: 226, 1974

15. Krueger SK, French JW, Forker AD, Caudill CC, Popp RL: Echocardiography in discrete subaortic stenosis. Circulation 59: 506, 1979

16. Weyman AE, Feigenbaum H, Hurwitz RA, Girod DA, Dillon JC, Chang S: Cross-sectional echocardiography in evaluating patients with discrete subaortic stenosis. Am J Cardiol 37: 358, 1976

17. Ten Cate FJ, Van Dorp WG, Hugenholtz PG, Roelandt J: Fixed subaortic stenosis: Value of echocardiography for diagnosis and differentiation between various types. Br Heart J 41: 159, 1979

18. Weyman AE, Caldwell RL, Hurwitz RA, Girod DA, Dillon JC, Feigenbaum H, Green D: Cross-sectional echocardiographic characterization of aortic obstruction. 1. Supravalvar aortic stenosis and aortic hypoplasia. Circulation 57: 491, 1978

19. Wing JP, Findlay WA, Sahn DJ, McDonald G, Allen HD, Goldberg SJ: Serial echocardiographic profiles in infants and children with coarctation of the aorta. Am J Cardiol 41: 1270, 1978

20. Sahn DJ, Allen HD, McDonald G, Goldberg SJ: Real-time cross-sectional echocardiographic diagnosis of coarctation of the aorta: A prospective study of echocardiographic-angiographic correlations. Circulation 56: 762, 1977

21. Weyman AE, Caldwell RL, Hurwitz RA, Girod DA, Dillon JC, Feigenbaum H, Green D: Cross-sectional echocardiographic detection of aortic obstruction. 2. Coarctation of the aorta. Circulation 57: 498, 1978

22. Ross AM, Pisarczyk MJ, Calabresi M: Echocardiographic and clinical correlations in systemic hypertension. J Clin Ultrasound 6: 95, 1978

23. Weyman AE, Hurwitz RA, Girod DA, Dillon JC, Feigenbaum H, Green D: Cross-sectional echocardiographic visualization of the stenotic pulmonary valve. Circulation 56: 769, 1977

CHAPTER 7

Ventricular Inflow Obstruction

LEFT VENTRICULAR INFLOW OBSTRUCTION

Congenital forms of left ventricular inflow obstruction include cor triatriatum, supravalvar mitral ring, congenital mitral valve stenosis, and parachute mitral valve deformity. The clinical manifestations of the various forms of left ventricular inflow obstruction are not helpful in determining the precise anatomic diagnosis, and the exact anatomy often is unclear even after a complete cardiac catheterization and cineangiography. The M-mode echocardiogram has been important in detecting the presence of left ventricular inflow obstruction[1-7] but has not proved useful in determining the exact anatomy.[8,9] In many instances, similar M-mode echocardiographic findings have been reported for very different anatomic defects.[1-7] Because of its ability to image the heart in several spatial planes, two-dimensional echocardiography can be used to determine the precise anatomy in cases of left ventricular inflow obstruction.[10]

Left Atrial Membranes

In patients with cor triatriatum and supravalvar mitral ring, a thin membrane can be seen stretching across the left atrium in the parasternal and apical long-axis views and in the apical and subcostal four-chamber views (Fig. 7-1). In real time, the left atrial membrane moves toward the mitral valve funnel in diastole and away from the mitral valve leaflets in systole. The exact attachments of the membrane are extremely difficult to image; however, in the long-axis views, the membrane stretches obliquely across the left atrium with extensions anterosuperiorly to the posterior aortic root and posteroinferiorly to the posterior left atrial wall. In the four-chamber views, the membrane is posi-

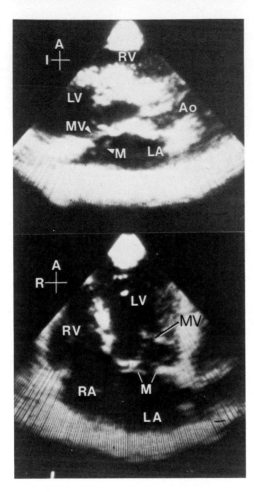

FIG. 7-1. Top. *Parasternal long-axis view from a 14-year-old male with a supravalvar mitral ring. A thin membrane (M) is seen stretching obliquely across the left atrium (LA) just above the mitral valve (MV). The mitral valve is thickened and the left atrium is enlarged. Because of associated dextroversion, the septum and left ventricular apex are not imaged clearly in this view. A, anterior; Ao, aorta; I, inferior; LV, left ventricle; RV, right ventricle.* **Bottom.** *Apical four-chamber view from the same patient. The membrane (M) is positioned horizontally in the left atrium (LA) just above the mitral valve (MV). The mitral valve echoes are much denser than the tricuspid valve echoes and the LA is enlarged. A, apex; LV, left ventricle; R, right; RA, right atrium; RV, right ventricle.*

tioned in a horizontal plane with extensions on the right to the interatrial septum and on the left to the lateral left atrial wall. Care must be taken not to confuse echoes arising from a thickened mitral valve annulus with echoes arising from a membrane in the mitral valve funnel. By directing careful attention to the gain and reject settings and to the motion of the echo in question, this misinterpretation can be avoided.

Cor triatriatum and supravalvar mitral ring can be differentiated by noting the position of the pulmonary veins and left atrial appendage relative to the membrane. In supravalvar mitral ring, the membrane is positioned adjacent to the mitral valve. In cor triatriatum, the membrane divides the left atrium into two chambers—a posterior, superior chamber that receives the pulmonary veins and an anterior, inferior chamber that gives rise to the left atrial append-age and communicates with the mitral valve. The division of the left atrium into these two chambers can be seen in the apical and subcostal four-chamber views.[11]

Patients with a left atrial membrane, especially those with a supravalvar mitral ring, may have an enlarged left atrium and a thickened mitral valve. In most patients with cor triatriatum, however, the mitral valve is normal.[8]

Mitral Valve Stenosis

In congenital mitral valve stenosis, the mitral valve leaflets appear thickened in all echocardiographic planes (Fig. 7-2). The leaflets move stiffly and exhibit a diminished diastolic excursion. There is usually prominent left atrial dilata-tion. Congenital mitral valve stenosis can occur with two normal papillary muscles or with papillary muscle fusion. With papillary muscle fusion, the mi-tral valve chordae are usually inserted into a single large papillary muscle. This so-called "parachute mitral valve deformity" is often associated with multiple left-sided obstructive lesions. The papillary muscle anatomy can be determined from the parasternal short-axis view through the left ventricle below the mitral valve leaflets. With congenital mitral valve stenosis and nor-mal papillary muscle anatomy, two equal-sized papillary muscles are seen in the circular left ventricle at approximately the 4 o'clock and 8 o'clock locations (Fig. 7-2). With congenital mitral valve stenosis caused by a parachute mitral valve deformity, a single large papillary muscle is seen arising from the poste-rior left ventricular wall (Fig. 7-3). Often, the single papillary muscle is seen projecting prominently into the left ventricle in the apical and subcostal views.

Several investigators have shown an excellent correlation between the mitral valve area measured from the parasternal short-axis view and the sever-ity of the mitral stenosis.[12,13] Cross-sectional echocardiography is also useful for quantitating the mitral valve area following mitral commissurotomy[14] and for evaluating the thin biologic tissue of the heterograft prosthetic mitral valve.[11]

RIGHT VENTRICULAR INFLOW OBSTRUCTION

Congenital tricuspid stenosis as an isolated defect is extremely rare. In the two patients we have studied with this defect, the tricuspid valve orifice in the apical and subcostal four-chamber views and in the parasternal and subcostal short-axis views was extremely small (Fig. 7-4). The tricuspid valve leaflets were diminutive, thickened, and moved stiffly. The right atrium was mark-edly enlarged and the atrial septum bulged toward the left (Fig. 7-5). The right ventricular cavity was small.

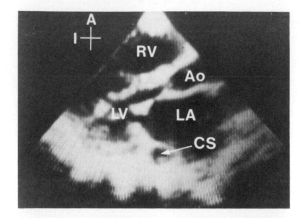

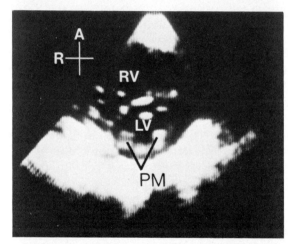

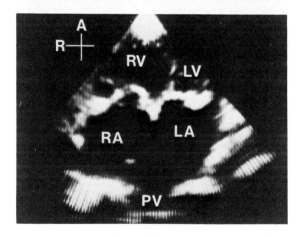

FIG. 7-2. Top. *Parasternal long-axis view from a 13-year-old female with congenital mitral valve stenosis. The mitral valve leaflets are thickened and the left atrium (LA) is enlarged. The right ventricle (RV) is enlarged because of long-standing pulmonary hypertension. The coronary sinus (CS) is enlarged because of a persistent left superior vena cava draining to the coronary sinus. A, anterior; Ao, aorta; I, inferior; LV, left ventricle.* **Middle.** *Parasternal short-axis view through the left ventricle (LV) below the mitral valve leaflets from the same patient. The presence of two normal papillary muscles (PM) excludes the possibility of a parachute mitral valve deformity. A, anterior; R, right; RV, right ventricle.* **Bottom.** *Apical four-chamber view from the same patient taken at the time of maximum diastolic opening of the mitral valve, which is severely limited compared to the tricuspid valve. The mitral valve is thickened and domed, and the left atrium (LA) is enlarged. The pulmonary veins (PV), right atrium (RA), and right ventricle (RV) are enlarged as a result of long-standing pulmonary hypertension. A, apex; LV, left ventricle; R, right.*

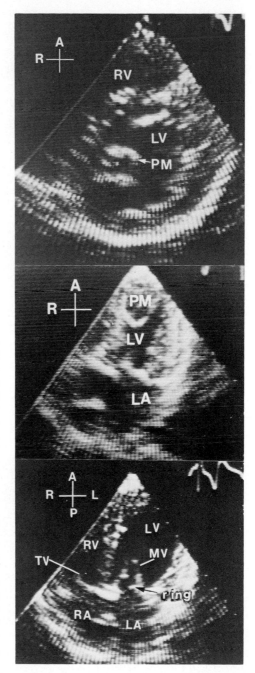

FIG. 7-3. Top. *Parasternal short-axis view through the left ventricle (LV) below the mitral valve leaflets from a patient with parachute mitral valve deformity. A single large papillary muscle (PM) is seen arising from the LV posterior wall. A, anterior; R, right; RV, right ventricle.* **Middle.** *Modified apical view from the same patient. The single papillary muscle (PM) is seen protruding into the left ventricle (LV). A, apex; LA, left atrium; R, right.* **Bottom.** *Apical four-chamber view from the same patient showing an associated defect—a supravalvar mitral ring. This patient also had Shone's complex (severe subaortic stenosis, coarctation of the aorta, and aortic valve stenosis). Note the conical shape of the mitral valve funnel caused by the insertion of all of the mitral valve (MV) chordae into a single papillary muscle (not seen in this view). A, anterior; L, left; LA, left atrium; LV, left ventricle; P, posterior; R, right; RA, right atrium; RV, right ventricle; TV, tricuspid valve.*

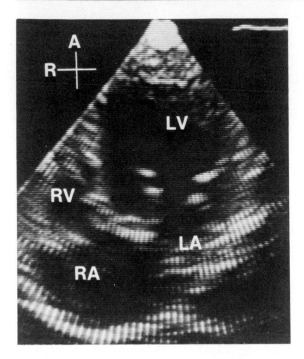

FIG. 7-4. *Apical   four-chamber view from a patient with isolated congenital tricuspid stenosis. The tricuspid valve orifice is extremely small and the leaflets are diminutive. The right atrium (RA) is enlarged and the atrial septum is bulging in a reverse manner toward the left. The right ventricle (RV) is small. A, apex; LA, left atrium; LV, left ventricle; R, right.*

FIG. 7-5. *Parasternal   long-axis view from a patient with congenital tricuspid valve stenosis. The right ventricle (RV) is small. The right atrium (RA) is so enlarged that it can be seen superior to the left atrium (LA) in this view. The interatrial septum bulges toward the LA. A, anterior; AO, aorta; I, inferior; LV, left ventricle.*

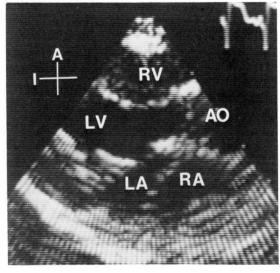

REFERENCES

1. Lundstrom N: Ultrasoundcardiographic studies of the mitral valve region in young infants with mitral atresia, mitral stenosis, hypoplasia of the left ventricle, and cor triatriatum. Circulation 45: 324, 1972

2. Chung KJ, Manning JA, Lipchik EO, Gramiak R, Mahoney EB: Isolated supravalvular stenosing ring of left atrium: Diagnosis before operation and successful surgical treatment. Chest 65: 25, 1974

3. Gibson DG, Honey M, Lennox SC: Cor triatriatum: Diagnosis by echocardiography. Br Heart J 36: 835, 1974

4. Nimura Y, Matsumoto M, Beppu S, Matsuo H, Sakakibara H, Abe H: Noninvasive preoperative diagnosis of cor triatriatum with ultrasonocardiotomogram and conventional echocardiogram. Am Heart J 88: 240, 1974

5. Moodie DS, Hagler DJ, Ritter DG: Cor triatriatum: Echocardiographic findings. Mayo Clin Proc 51: 289, 1976

6. Cooperberg P, Hazell S, Ashmore PG: Parachute accessory anterior mitral valve leaflet causing left ventricular outflow tract obstruction. Circulation 53: 908, 1976

7. Canedo MI, Stefadouros MA, Frank MJ, Moore HV, Cundey DW: Echocardiographic features of cor triatriatum. Am J Cardiol 40: 615, 1977

8. LaCorte M, Harada K, Williams RG: Echocardiographic features of congenital left ventricular inflow obstruction. Circulation 54: 562, 1976

9. Driscoll DJ, Gutgesell HP, McNamara DG: Echocardiographic features of congenital mitral stenosis. Am J Cardiol 42: 259, 1978

10. Snider AR, Rogé CL, Schiller NB, Silverman NH: Congenital left ventricular inflow obstruction evaluated by two-dimensional echocardiography. Circulation 61:848, 1980

11. Goldberg SJ, Allen HD, Sahn DJ: Pediatric and Adolescent Echocardiography: A Handbook. Chicago, Year Book Medical Publishers, 1980

12. Henry WL, Griffith JM, Michaelis LL, McIntosh CL, Morrow AG, Epstein SE: Measurement of mitral orifice area in patients with mitral valve disease by real-time, two-dimensional echocardiography. Circulation 51: 287, 1975

13. Nichol PM, Gilbert BW, Kisslo JA: Two-dimensional echocardiographic assessment of mitral stenosis. Circulation 55: 120, 1977

14. Heger JJ, Wann LS, Weyman AE, Dillon JC, Feigenbaum H: Long-term changes in mitral valve area after successful mitral commissurotomy. Circulation 59: 443, 1979

CHAPTER 8

Other Acyanotic Lesions

MITRAL VALVE PROLAPSE/TRICUSPID VALVE PROLAPSE

Mitral valve prolapse is a common condition in children that occurs as an isolated defect or in association with congenital heart disease, straight back syndrome, skeletal abnormalities such as pectus excavatum, or connective tissue disorders such as Marfan syndrome. The degree of mitral valve prolapse is affected by many factors including ventricular size and shape, chordal length, leaflet length, and leaflet morphology.[1] Various M-mode echocardiographic patterns ranging from late systolic dipping to holosystolic hammocking have been described in patients with mitral valve prolapse.[2-4] Two-dimensional echocardiographic studies suggest that this variety of M-mode echocardiographic patterns results from examining different portions of the mitral valve. On the two-dimensional echocardiographic examination, most cases of mitral valve prolapse involve both the anterior and posterior mitral valve leaflets.[5,6]

In the parasternal and apical long-axis views in patients with a normal mitral valve, both mitral valve leaflets arch slightly toward each other in systole and the mitral apparatus descends anteriorly and inferiorly. During systole, a slight posterior curvature of the anterior mitral valve leaflet is normal.[7] In the long-axis views in systole in patients with mitral valve prolapse, superior arching of the midportions of the anterior and posterior mitral valve leaflets above the level of the mitral ring occurs so that the leaflets billow into the left atrium (Figs. 8-1 and 8-2)[5-7] The leaflet displacement in mitral valve prolapse occurs mainly in a superior direction toward the left atrium; however, a slight posterior displacement is also common. Other common findings in patients with mitral valve prolapse include (1) a more posterior position of the coaptation

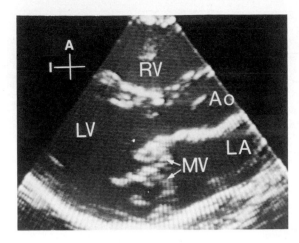

FIG. 8-1. *Parasternal long-axis view from a patient with isolated mitral valve (MV) prolapse. The midportions of both mitral valve leaflets are arched superior to the mitral ring into the left atrium (LA). A, anterior; Ao, aorta; I, inferior; LV, left ventricle; RV, right ventricle.*

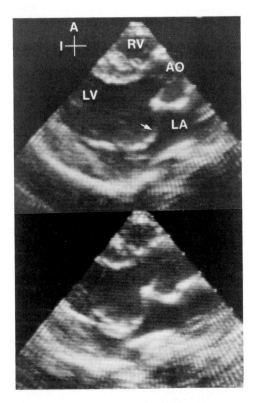

FIG. 8-2. *Parasternal long-axis views in early (**top**) and late (**bottom**) systole from a patient with mitral valve prolapse. The anterior mitral valve leaflet (arrow) is large and redundant. Both leaflets arch superior and posterior into the left atrium (LA). The coaptation point of the mitral leaflets is more posterior than usual. The aorta (AO) and sinuses of Valsalva are dilated. A, anterior; I, inferior; LV, left ventricle; RV, right ventricle.*

point of the mitral leaflets, (2) systolic curling of the mitral ring on the adjacent myocardium, and (3) large, redundant anterior mitral valve leaflet with a whiplike motion during early diastole.[7] In addition, the myxomatous mitral valve degeneration that is present in patients with mitral valve prolapse causes the mitral leaflets to appear thickened and shaggy on the two-dimensional echocardiogram. Although the apical and subcostal four-chamber views can be used to detect billowing of the mitral leaflets into the left atrium of patients with significant mitral valve prolapse (Fig. 8-3), the four-chamber views may not be as sensitive as the long-axis view for detecting mild mitral valve prolapse with predominantly superior displacement of the mitral leaflets (Fig. 8-4).

Using M-mode echocardiograms derived from the two-dimensional image, Sahn and colleagues have shown that a variety of patterns of mitral valve prolapse can be obtained from the same patient by sampling different portions of the mitral leaflets.[5,6] Patterns suggesting more severe, holosystolic prolapse were obtained from the superiorly arched midportions of the mitral leaflets. M-mode echocardiograms taken from the free edges of the mitral leaflets usually showed less severe evidence of mitral prolapse and corresponded more closely with the findings on the physical examination.

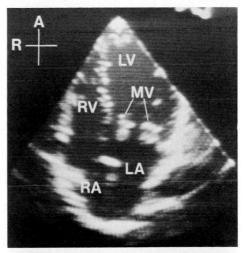

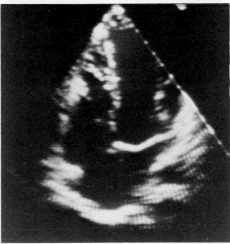

FIG. 8-3. *Apical four-chamber views in diastole* (**top**) *and systole* (**bottom**) *from a patient with mitral valve prolapse. The mitral valve (MV) leaflets are thickened and shaggy and are displaced into the left atrium (LA) in systole. A, apex; LV, left ventricle; R, right; RA, right atrium; RV, right ventricle.*

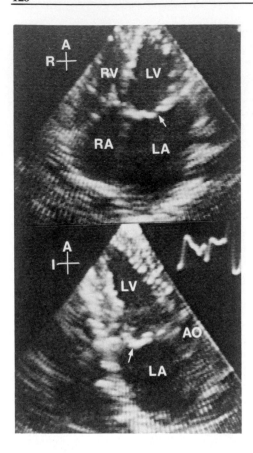

FIG. 8-4. Top. *Apical four-chamber view from a patient with significant mitral valve prolapse and mitral insufficiency. A slight posterior displacement (arrow) of the mitral leaflets into the left atrium (LA) is seen. The left atrium and left ventricle (LV) are dilated. A, apex; R, right; RA, right atrium; RV, right ventricle.* **Bottom.** *Apical long-axis view from the same patient. The mitral valve prolapse, which occurs in a predominantly superior direction (arrow), is more obvious in the apical long-axis view. The mitral valve is thickened and the left atrium (LA) and left ventricle (LV) are dilated. A, anterior; AO, aorta; I, inferior.*

Most children with isolated mitral valve prolapse have minimal or no evidence of mitral regurgitation. In these patients, the left atrium and left ventricle are of normal size or are minimally enlarged. When significant mitral regurgitation is present, left atrial and left ventricular dilatation can be seen on the two-dimensional echocardiogram (Fig. 8-4). Many patients with mitral valve prolapse and no physical stigmata of Marfan syndrome have enlargement of the aortic root and dilatation of the sinuses of Valsalva (Fig. 8-2).[5,6] Whether or not these patients have a form of connective tissue disorder remains to be determined.

Several studies have reported that from 21 to 52 percent of patients with mitral valve prolapse also have tricuspid valve prolapse.[8-10] Those patients with tricuspid valve prolapse usually have a more severe form of mitral valve prolapse. In the long-axis view of the right ventricle and the apical four-chamber view in patients with tricuspid valve prolapse, both tricuspid leaflets arch superior to the tricuspid ring into the right atrium (Fig. 8-5). In those patients with tricuspid valve prolapse and significant tricuspid insufficiency, right atrial and right ventricular enlargement are usually present.

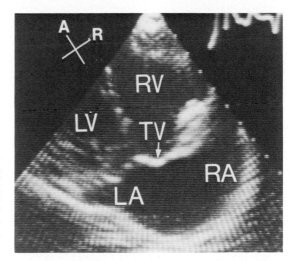

FIG. 8-5. *Long-axis view through the right ventricle (RV) in a patient with mitral and tricuspid valve (TV) prolapse. The tricuspid leaflets arch superior above the tricuspid ring into the right atrium (RA). A, apex; LA, left atrium; LV, left ventricle; R, right.*

HEART DISEASE IN MARFAN SYNDROME

A high percentage of patients with Marfan syndrome have mitral valve prolapse and/or aortic root dilatation. These defects are caused by disruption of the normal architecture of connective tissue and, when severe, lead to aortic and mitral insufficiency.[11-13]

Aortic root dilatation, which can be seen in the parasternal and apical long-axis views, can involve the entire aortic root (Fig. 8-6) or can involve one of the sinuses of Valsalva to a greater extent (Fig. 8-7). If significant aortic insufficiency occurs, the left ventricle will be dilated.

The appearance of mitral valve prolapse on the two-dimensional echocardiogram was discussed in the previous section. Patients with Marfan syndrome usually have a severe form of mitral valve prolapse.

TUMORS, CLOTS, FOREIGN BODIES

In adults, the most common primary cardiac tumor is the left atrial myxoma. In pediatric patients, left atrial myxomas are rare, and most primary cardiac tumors are solid, nonmobile tumors such as sarcomas, lipomas, rhabdomyomas, and fibromas.[14] On the two-dimensional echocardiogram, left atrial myxomas appear as a mass of echoes behind the mitral valve that move with the direction of blood flow. Frequently, the myxoma passes through the mitral valve in diastole. Intracavitary tumors may be difficult to distinguish from thrombus by two-dimensional echocardiography. Also, tumor echoes can be difficult to distinguish from artifactual noise and may be obliterated by reject settings that are too high.[1]

Nonmobile, solid tumors in children are usually intramural tumors such as fibromas, rhabdomyomas, or sarcomas. On the two-dimensional echocar-

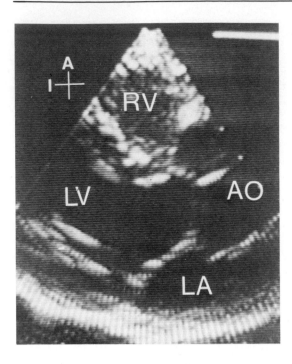

FIG. 8-6. *Parasternal long-axis view from a patient with Marfan syndrome. There is uniform dilatation of the entire aortic root (AO). A, anterior; I, inferior; LA, left atrium; LV, left ventricle; RV, right ventricle.*

diogram, these tumors appear as a localized, excessive thickening in the cardiac wall and may be associated with cavity obliteration (Figs. 8-8 to 8-10). Some solid tumors, especially fibromas, may protrude into the ventricular cavity. Two-dimensional echocardiography allows a better appreciation of the size of the tumor and its encroachment on surrounding cardiac structures.

Rhabdomyoma, the commonest cardiac tumor in infants, is frequently associated with tuberous sclerosis. The tumor usually consists of multiple small nodules in the left ventricular wall but may also involve the right ventricular wall and the valves themselves.[14] In several patients with tuberous sclerosis and rhabdomyoma whom we have examined by two-dimensional echocardiography, the tumor nodules were frequently found in the left ventricular papillary muscles (Figs. 8-11 and 8-12).

Occasionally, extracardiac tumors in the pericardium or anterior mediastinum can be detected by two-dimensional echocardiography (Fig. 8-13). Often, these tumors compress the right ventricular outflow tract and pulmonary artery. Mediastinal tumors frequently exhibit nonuniform echo reflectance because of cystic areas present within the tumor.

Intracardiac thrombi can occur in the atria, in the ventricles, or within the atrioventricular valve apparatus. Thrombi that are attached to the atrioventricular valve apparatus can be difficult to distinguish from valvar vegetations. Left atrial thrombi are frequently seen in patients with conditions causing left atrial dilatation such as mitral stenosis or atrial fibrillation (Fig. 8-14). As with atrial myxomas, these thrombi can be difficult to distinguish from echocardio-

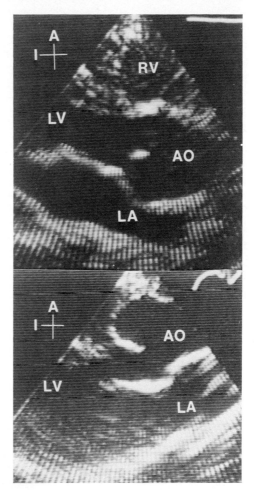

FIG. 8-7. **Top.** *Parasternal long-axis view from a patient with Marfan syndrome and aortic root (AO) enlargement. The posterior sinus of Valsalva is dilated to a greater extent than the other sinuses of Valsalva. A, anterior; I, inferior; LA, left atrium; LV, left ventricle; RV, right ventricle.* **Bottom.** *Parasternal long-axis view from a patient with Marfan syndrome and aortic root (AO) dilatation. The right sinus of Valsalva is dilated to a greater extent than the other sinuses of Valsalva. A, anterior; I, inferior; LA, left atrium; LV, left ventricle.*

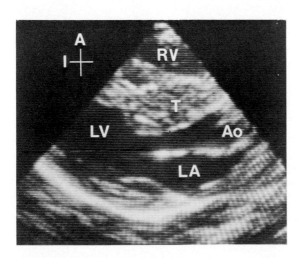

FIG. 8-8. *Parasternal long-axis view from an 11-year-old male with a solid, nonpedunculated tumor (T). The tumor extends from the septum to above the level of the aortic (Ao) valve and projects into the right ventricular (RV) outflow tract. The tumor is also encroaching on the left ventricular (LV) outflow tract. A, anterior; I, inferior; LA, left atrium.*

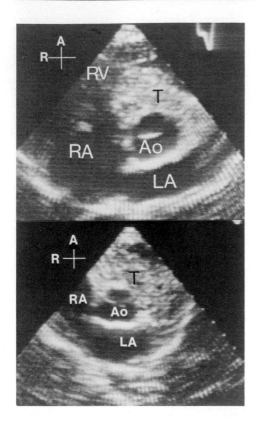

FIG. 8-9. *Parasternal short axis views from the same patient as in Fig. 8-8. The tumor (T) encircles the aorta (Ao) and is encroaching upon the right ventricular (RV) cavity. The tumor also appears to encircle the coronary arteries. A, anterior; LA, left atrium; R, right; RA, right atrium.*

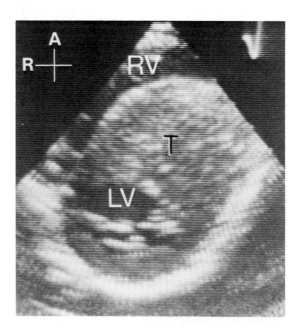

FIG. 8-10. *Parasternal short-axis view from the same patient as in Figs. 8-8 and 8-9. The tumor (T) appears as a localized thickening in the cardiac wall with encroachment on the cavities of the right ventricle (RV) and left ventricle (LV). A, anterior; R, right.*

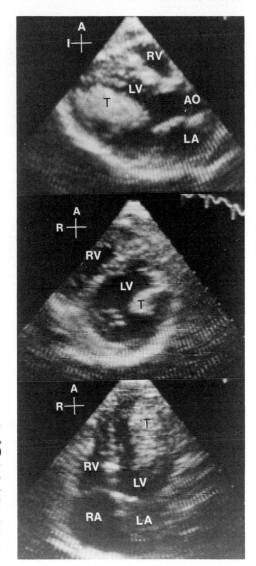

FIG. 8-11. *Parasternal long-axis view* (**top**), *parasternal short-axis* (**middle**), *and apical four-chamber view* (**bottom**) *from a patient with tuberous sclerosis and rhabdomyoma. The rhabdomyoma is a solid, intramural tumor (T) involving the left ventricular (LV) posterior wall and the anterolateral papillary muscle. A, anterior; AO, aorta; I, inferior; LA, left atrium; R, right; RA, right atrium; RV, right ventricle.*

graphic noise and can be obliterated by high reject settings. We have detected right heart thrombi by two-dimensional echocardiography in two patients following prolonged parenteral hyperalimentation (Figs. 8-15 and 8-16).

Vegetations in patients with bacterial endocarditis appear on two-dimensional echocardiography as shaggy, irregular structures with oscillating motion.[15,16] Vegetations can be seen attached to valves, the rims of ventricular septal defects, or prosthetic patches. Small vegetations may be missed on the two-dimensional echocardiographic examination.

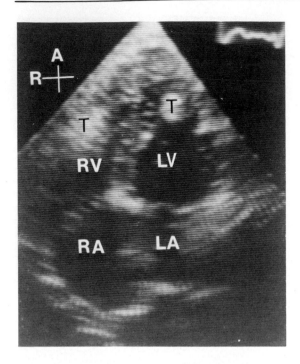

FIG. 8-12. *Apical four-chamber view from a patient with tuberous sclerosis and multiple rhabdomyoma. The rhabdomyoma are small, nodular tumors (T) in the walls of the right ventricle (RV) and left ventricle (LV). A, apex; LA, left atrium; R, right; RA, right atrium.*

Probably the most common foreign bodies that embolize to the heart are catheter tips. These catheters may break off during catheterization, during removal of monitoring lines in postoperative patients, or from shunts placed in hydrocephalic patients. The two-dimensional examination is useful for determining the exact location of the embolized catheter tip. On the two-dimensional examination, catheters give rise to linear, highly reflective echoes (Fig. 8-17). An M-mode echocardiogram taken through the catheter on the two-dimensional image shows two dense echoes separated by an echo-free space. The two dense echoes arise from the catheter walls and the echo-free space represents the catheter lumen.

THYMUS

In the parasternal long- and short-axis views and the suprasternal notch long-axis view in many infants and children, homogeneous echoes arising from the thymus can be seen anterior to the right ventricular outflow tract, ascending aorta, and main pulmonary artery (Fig. 8-18). The thymus has the reflectance properties of tissue, and, unlike some mediastinal tumors, does not cause cardiac compression.

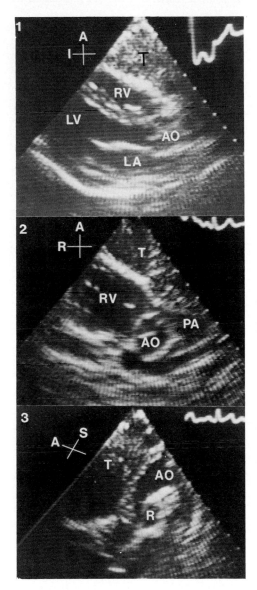

FIG. 8-13. *Parasternal long-axis view (1), parasternal short-axis view (2) and suprasternal notch long-axis view (3) from a patient with a mediastinal tumor (T). The tumor is compressing the right ventricle (RV), pulmonary artery (PA), and ascending aorta (AO). The echoes arising from the tumor are nonuniform in density because of cystic areas within the tumor. A, anterior; I, inferior; LA, left atrium; LV, left ventricle: R, right; S, superior.*

LEFT SUPERIOR VENA CAVA DRAINING TO THE CORONARY SINUS

A persistent left superior vena cava draining to the coronary sinus occurs in approximately 0.5 percent of the normal population and in approximately 3 to 10 percent of patients with congenital heart disease.[17] The increased blood

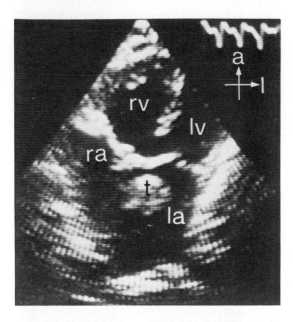

FIG. 8-14. *Apical four-chamber view from a patient with double outlet right ventricle (rv), mitral stenosis, and a large thrombus (t) in the left atrium (la). The right ventricle is thickened and apex forming and the left atrium is enlarged. A large ventricular septal defect is present. a, apex; l, left; lv, left ventricle; ra, right atrium.*

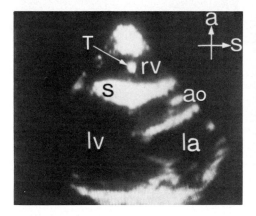
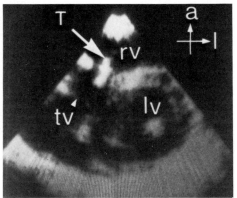

FIG. 8-15. *Parasternal long-axis view* (**left**) *and parasternal short-axis view* (**right**) *from a patient with a right ventricular thrombus (T) that formed following prolonged parenteral hyperalimentation. a, anterior; ao, aorta; l, left; la, left atrium; lv, left ventricle; rv, right ventricle; s, superior; S, septum; tv, tricuspid valve.*

flow to the coronary sinus causes enlargement of the coronary sinus that can be detected in several echocardiographic views.[18] In the parasternal long-axis view, the coronary sinus is seen in cross section as a discrete circular structure adjacent and slightly superior to the posterior mitral valve leaflet (see Fig. 4-7). In the parasternal short-axis view, the coronary sinus is seen at the level of the anterior mitral valve leaflet just below the standard short-axis view

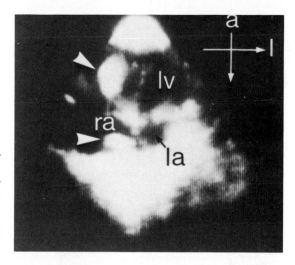

FIG. 8-16. *Apical four-chamber view from an infant with right atrial (ra) and right ventricular thrombi (arrows) following prolonged parenteral hyperalimentation for a gastroschisis. a, apex; l, left; la, left atrium; lv, left ventricle.*

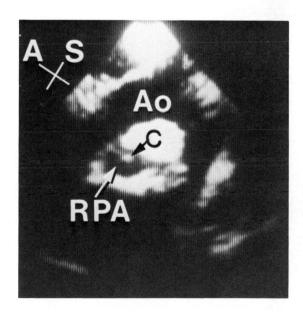

FIG. 8-17. *Suprasternal notch long-axis view from a patient in whom the tip of a shunt placed for hydrocephalus broke off. On the two-dimensional echocardiogram, the catheter (C) was found lodged in the right pulmonary artery (RPA). A, anterior; Ao, aorta; S, superior.*

through the aorta. In this view, the coronary sinus appears as a crescent-shaped structure posterior to the left ventricle and continuous with the right atrium (see Fig. 4-8). In the apical four-chamber view, the coronary sinus appears as an oval-shaped structure along the lateral border of the left atrium (see Fig. 4-9). Following saline contrast injections into a left arm vein, the coronary sinus fills first with contrast echoes. Next, the right atrium and right ventricle opacify due to forward flow from the coronary sinus.

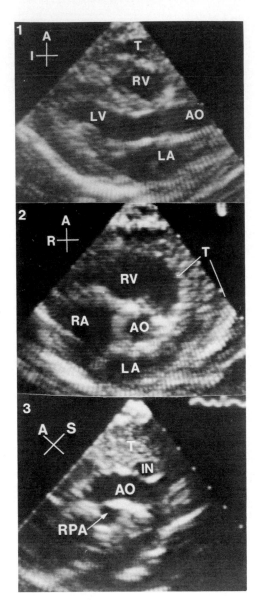

FIG. 8-18. *Parasternal long-axis view (1), parasternal short-axis view (2), and suprasternal notch long-axis view (3) from an infant with a normal thymus (T). The homogeneous echoes arising from the thymus have the same reflectance as tissue and are seen anterior to the right ventricle (RV) and ascending aorta (AO). A, anterior; I, inferior; IN, innominate vein; LA, left atrium; LV, left ventricle; R, right; RA, right atrium; RPA, right pulmonary artery; S, superior.*

In some patients, the left superior vena cava can be visualized directly in the suprasternal notch short-axis view. In patients with both a right and a left superior vena cava, these vessels are seen along both sides of the transverse aorta. An innominate vein connecting the superior venae cavae may be present or absent. In patients with a left superior vena cava and absence of the right superior vena cava, the superior vena cava is seen along the left side of the transverse aorta (Fig. 8-19). No vessel is present along the right side of the transverse aorta. The right innominate vein courses from right to left above the transverse aorta. The usual pattern of a left innominate vein coursing from left to right superior to the transverse aorta is absent. The left superior vena cava can be imaged more easily by tilting the transducer toward the patient's left in the suprasternal notch short-axis view.

IDIOPATHIC HYPERTROPHIC SUBAORTIC STENOSIS

Classic idiopathic hypertrophic subaortic stenosis is a hypertrophic cardio-myopathy characterized by disproportionate ventricular septal thickening and

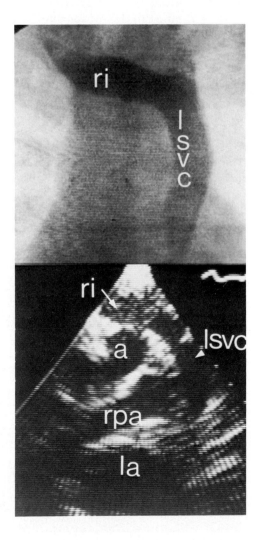

FIG. 8-19. *Frame from a cineangiogram* (**top**) *and suprasternal notch short-axis view* (**bottom**) *from a patient with absence of the right superior vena cava and a persistent left superior vena cava (lsvc) connecting to the coronary sinus. The right innominate vein (ri) courses from right to left superior to the transverse aorta (a). la, left atrium; rpa, right pulmonary artery.*

marked septal cardiac muscle cell disorganization.[19] The disorder is usually inherited as an autosomal dominant pattern with complete penetration. The M-mode echocardiographic features of idiopathic hypertrophic subaortic stenosis include: (1) septal/left ventricular free wall ratio of 1.3 or greater, (2) systolic anterior motion of the mitral valve, and (3) midsystolic closure of the aortic valve.[20-23] The two-dimensional echocardiogram has allowed a better appreciation of the extent of myocardial involvement and the mechanism of obstruction in these patients.[23-25]

On the two-dimensional echocardiogram of patients with idiopathic hypertrophic subaortic stenosis, the ventricular septum is usually considerably thicker than the left ventricular posterior wall (Figs. 8-20 to 8-23). Although the entire left ventricle can be hypertrophic, the ventricular septum is usually involved to a far greater extent (Fig. 8-22). Hypertrophy of the ventricular septum is greatest in the midportion of the septum and does not usually involve the area of the membranous septum. As on the M-mode echocardiogram, the true right surface of the septum can be difficult to resolve on the two-dimensional study.

The obstruction in idiopathic hypertrophic subaortic stenosis appears to be caused by abnormal apposition in systole between the anterior mitral valve leaflet and the hypertrophied septum. It is believed that the rapid flow velocity in the left ventricular outflow tract in systole creates a Venturi effect causing the mitral valve leaflet tip and chordae to be sucked into the outflow tract.[23] This systolic anterior motion of the mitral valve can be seen in the long- and short-axis views. In general, patients with no evidence of systolic anterior motion of the mitral valve have no obstruction at rest; patients in

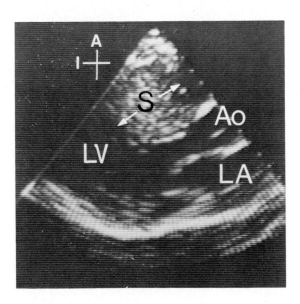

FIG. 8-20. *Parasternal long-axis view from a patient with idiopathic hypertrophic subaortic stenosis. There is marked thickening of the midportion of the septum (S). A, anterior; Ao, aorta; I, inferior; LA, left atrium; LV, left ventricle.*

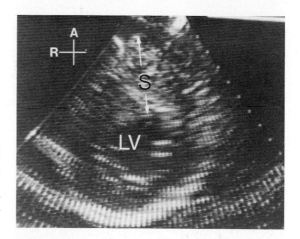

FIG. 8-21. *Parasternal short-axis view through the left ventricle (LV) from a patient with idiopathic hypertrophic subaortic stenosis. The septum (S) is far thicker than the left ventricular posterior wall. A, anterior; R, right.*

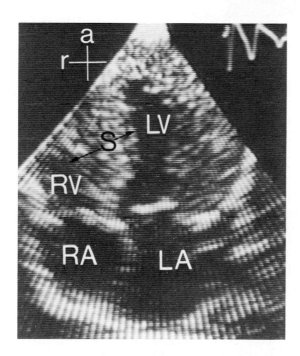

FIG. 8-22. *Apical four-chamber view from a patient with idiopathic hypertrophic subaortic stenosis. The entire left ventricle (LV) is hypertrophic; however, the septum (S) is involved to a far greater extent. a, apex; LA, left atrium; r, right; RA, right atrium; RV, right ventricle.*

whom the mitral valve just touches the septum have mild obstruction; and patients in whom the mitral valve is plastered against the septum have severe obstruction.[1]

Occasionally, mitral valve prolapse can be seen on the two-dimensional echocardiogram in patients with idiopathic hypertrophic subaortic stenosis. Mitral insufficiency, which can occur with significant hypertrophic cardio-

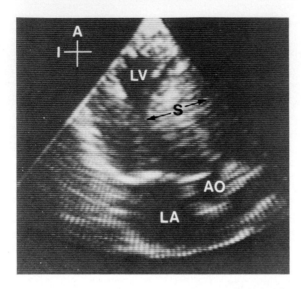

FIG. 8-23. *Apical long-axis view from a patient with idiopathic hypertrophic subaortic stenosis. The midportion of the septum (S) is markedly thickened. The membranous septum is of normal thickness. A, anterior; AO, aorta; I, inferior; LA, left atrium; LV, left ventricle.*

myopathy,[26] can lead to left atrial enlargement on the two-dimensional examination.

The two-dimensional echocardiogram is especially useful in the assessment of patients who have undergone septal myectomy.[27] The area of surgical enlargement of the left ventricular outflow tract, which usually has an irregular shape, can be better visualized by two-dimensional echocardiography (Fig. 8-24).

We believe that echocardiographic examination should be performed on the family members of patients with idiopathic hypertrophic subaortic stenosis because of the 50 percent inheritance rate. Family members can have obstructive or silent (nonobstructive) forms of the disease.

INFANT OF DIABETIC MOTHER CARDIOMYOPATHY

Many infants of diabetic mothers have a cardiomyopathy characterized by generalized cardiac hypertrophy with disproportionate septal thickening.[28,29] On the two-dimensional sector scan, these patients can have the same appearance as patients with idiopathic hypertrophic subaortic stenosis (Fig. 8-25). The history of diabetes in the mother helps differentiate this condition from idiopathic hypertrophic subaortic stenosis. In addition, the two-dimensional echocardiogram often shows hypertrophy of the right ventricular anterior wall and left ventricular posterior wall with encroachment on both ventricular cavities. The disease is self-limited and usually resolves in 6 to 8 months.

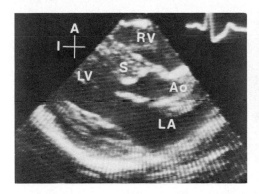
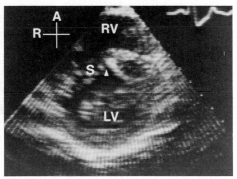

FIG. 8-24. *Parasternal long- (left) and short- (right) axis views from a patient with idiopathic hypertrophic subaortic stenosis following myectomy. The area of surgical enlargement of the left ventricular (LV) outflow tract (arrow) is irregular in shape. A, anterior; Ao, aorta; I, inferior; LA, left atrium; R, right; RV, right ventricle; S, septum.*

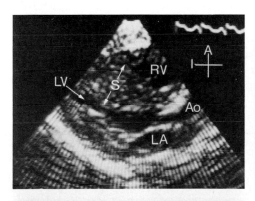
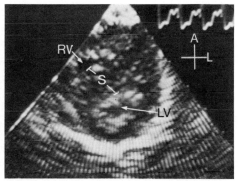

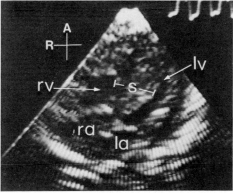

FIG. 8-25. *Parasternal long-axis view (left), parasternal short-axis view (right), and apical four-chamber view (left-bottom) from a newborn infant of a diabetic mother. There is generalized cardiac hypertrophy with involvement of the septum (S) to a far greater degree. The cardiac hypertrophy is encroaching on the cavities of the right and left ventricles (RV and LV). A, anterior; Ao, aorta, I, inferior; L, left; LA, left atrium; R, right; RA, right atrium.*

RHEUMATIC HEART DISEASE

Rheumatic heart disease results most commonly in aortic or mitral insufficiency. On the two-dimensional echocardiogram in patients with significant mitral insufficiency, the left ventricle is enlarged and hyperdynamic and the left atrium is dilated (Fig. 8-26). Frequently, the mitral valve leaflets are densely reflective. In some patients, mitral prolapse can be seen in association with rheumatic mitral insufficiency.[30] In patients with long-standing rheumatic mitral valve disease, there may be signs of concomitant mitral stenosis such as doming and restricted diastolic opening (Fig. 8-26). There are no specific echocardiographic features that distinguish rheumatic mitral insufficiency from nonrheumatic mitral insufficiency. Other structural defects that cause mitral insufficiency such as papillary muscle anomalies, mitral valve prolapse, and cleft anterior mitral valve leaflet should be sought on the two-dimensional echocardiographic examination.

In patients with rheumatic aortic insufficiency, the left ventricle is usually dilated and hypercontractile. In the parasternal short-axis view, the edges of the rheumatic aortic valve cusps are frequently thickened and fail to close completely in diastole. We have seen several patients with rheumatic aortic insufficiency and prolapse of an aortic valve cusp (Fig. 8-27). There are no specific echocardiographic features that distinguish rheumatic aortic insufficiency from nonrheumatic aortic insufficiency. Other defects causing aortic

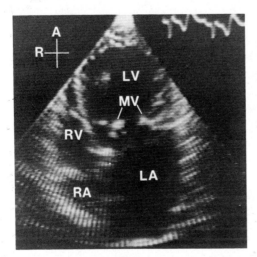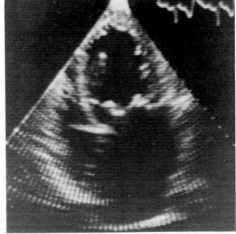

FIG. 8-26. *Apical four-chamber views in diastole* (**left**) *and systole* (**right**) *from a patient with severe rheumatic mitral insufficiency and mild mitral stenosis. The left atrium (LA) and left ventricle (LV) are enlarged. The mitral valve (MV) is thickened and domed in diastole. In systole, the mitral valve arches toward the left atrium. A, apex; R, right; RA, right atrium; RV, right ventricle.*

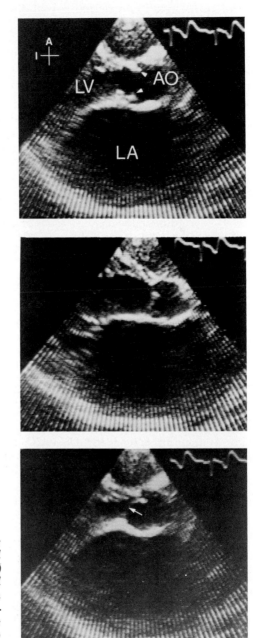

FIG. 8-27. *Parasternal long-axis views from a patient with rheumatic aortic and mitral insufficiency. The left atrium (LA) is enlarged. In systole (**top**), the thickened aortic (AO) valve leaflets are seen (arrows). In diastole (**middle and bottom**), the posterior aortic cusp prolapses into the left ventricular (LV) outflow tract (arrow). A, anterior; I, inferior.*

insufficiency such as bicuspid aortic valve, aortico–left ventricular tunnel, and supracristal ventricular septal defect with a prolapsed aortic cusp should be sought on the two-dimensional echocardiographic examination.

REFERENCES

1. Goldberg SJ, Allen HD, Sahn DJ: Pediatric and Adolescent Echocardiography. Chicago, Year Book Medical Publishers, 1980
2. Dillon JC, Haine CL, Chang S, Feigenbaum H: Use of echocardiography in patients with prolapsed mitral valve. Circulation 43: 503, 1971
3. Popp RL, Brown OR, Silverman JF, Harrison DC: Echocardiographic abnormalities in the mitral valve prolapse syndrome. Circulation 49: 428, 1974
4. DeMaria AN, King JF, Bogren HG, Lies JE, Mason DT: The variable spectrum of echocardiographic manifestations of mitral valve prolapse. Circulation 50: 33, 1974
5. Sahn DJ, Allen HD, Goldberg SJ, Friedman WF: Mitral valve prolapse in children: A problem defined by real-time cross-sectional echocardiography. Circulation 53: 651, 1976
6. Sahn DJ, Wood J, Allen HD, Peoples W, Goldberg SJ: Echocardiographic spectrum of mitral valve motion in children with and without mitral valve prolapse: The nature of false positive diagnosis. Am J Cardiol 39: 422, 1977
7. Gilbert BW, Schatz RA, Von Ramm OT, Behar VS, Kisslo JA: Mitral valve prolapse: Two-dimensional echocardiographic and angiographic correlations. Circulation 54: 716, 1976
8. Gooch AS, Maranhao V, Scampardonis G, Cha SD, Yang SS: Prolapse of both mitral and tricuspid leaflets in systolic murmur-click syndrome. N Engl J Med 287; 1218, 1972
9. Werner JA, Schiller NB, Prasquier R: Occurrence and significance of echocardiographically demonstrated tricuspid valve prolapse. Am Heart J 96: 180, 1978
10. Morgenroth J, Jones RH, Chen CC, Naito M: Two-dimensional echocardiography in mitral, aortic and tricuspid valve prolapse: The clinical problem, cardiac nuclear imaging considerations and a proposed standard for diagnosis. Am J Cardiol 46: 1164, 1980
11. Brown OR, De Mots H, Kloster FE, Roberts A, Menashe VD, Beals RK: Aortic root dilatation and mitral valve prolapse in Marfan's syndrome: An echocardiographic study. Circulation 52: 651, 1975
12. Spangler RD, Nora JJ, Lortscher RH, Wolfe RR, Okin JT: Echocardiography in Marfan's syndrome. Chest 69: 72, 1976
13. Freed C, Schiller NB: Echocardiographic findings in Marfan's syndrome. West J Med 126: 87, 1977
14. Nadas AS, Ellison RC: Cardiac tumors in infancy. Am J Cardiol 21: 363, 1968
15. Kisslo J, Von Ramm OT, Haney R, Jones R, Juk SS, Behar VS: Echocardiographic evaluation of tricuspid valve endocarditis: An M-mode and two-dimensional study. Am J Cardiol 38: 502, 1976
16. Mintz GS, Kotler MN, Segal BL, Parry WR: Comparison of two-dimensional and M-mode echocardiography in the evaluation of patients with infective endocarditis. Am J Cardiol 43: 738, 1979
17. Mantini E, Grondin CM, Lillehei CW, Edwards JE: Congenital anomalies involving the coronary sinus. Circulation 33: 317, 1966

18. Snider AR, Ports TA, Silverman NH: Venous anomalies of the coronary sinus: Detection by M-mode, two-dimensional and contrast echocardiography. Circulation 60: 721, 1979

19. Maron BJ, Roberts WC: Quantitative analysis of cardiac muscle cell disorganization in the ventricular septum of patients with hypertrophic cardiomyopathy. Circulation 59: 689, 1979

20. Shah PM, Gramiak R, Kramer DH: Ultrasound location of left ventricular outflow obstruction in hypertrophic obstructive cardiomyopathy. Circulation 40: 3, 1969

21. Popp RL, Harrison DC: Ultrasound in the diagnosis and evaluation of therapy of idiopathic hypertrophic subaortic stenosis. Circulation 40: 905, 1969

22. Henry WL, Clark CE, Epstein SE: Asymmetric septal hypertrophy: Echocardiographic identification of the pathognomonic anatomic abnormality of IHSS. Circulation 47: 225, 1973

23. Henry WL, Clark CE, Griffith JM, Epstein SE: Mechanism of left ventricular outflow obstruction in patients with obstructive asymmetric septal hypertrophy (idiopathic hypertrophic subaortic stenosis). Am J Cardiol 35: 337, 1975

24. Cohen MV, Teichholz LE, Gorlin R: B-scan ultrasonography in idiopathic hypertrophic subaortic stenosis. Study of left ventricular outflow tract and mechanisms of obstruction. Br Heart J 38: 595, 1976

25. Martin RP, Rakowski H, French J, Popp RL: Idiopathic hypertrophic subaortic stenosis viewed by wide-angle, phased-array echocardiography. Circulation 59: 1206, 1979

26. Pridie RB, Oakley CM: Mechanism of mitral regurgitation in hypertrophic obstructive cardiomyopathy. Br Heart J 32: 203, 1970

27. Schapira JN, Stemple DR, Martin RP, Rakowski H, Stinson EB, Popp RL: Single and two-dimensional echocardiographic visualization of the effects of septal myectomy in idiopathic hypertrophic subaortic stenosis. Circulation 58: 850, 1978

28. Gutgesell HP, Speer ME, Rosenberg HS: Characterization of the cardiomyopathy in infants of diabetic mothers. Circulation 61: 441, 1980

29. Mace S, Hirschfeld SS, Riggs T, Fanaroff AA, Merkatz IR, Franklin W: Echocardiographic abnormalities in infants of diabetic mothers. J Pediatr 95: 1013, 1979

30. Steinfeld L, Dimich I, Rappaport H, Baron M: Late systolic murmur of rheumatic insufficiency. Am J Cardiol 35: 397, 1975

CHAPTER 9

Conditions with Override of the Ventricular Septum by the Systemic Artery

The echocardiographic finding of a dilated systemic artery overriding the ventricular septum is a feature of a group of conotruncal abnormalities, including tetralogy of Fallot, pulmonary atresia with a ventricular septal defect, persistent truncus arteriosus, and double outlet right ventricle. Besides anterior discontinuity, these four conotruncal defects share the following M-mode echocardiographic findings: (1) increased right ventricular diameter, (2) thickening of the right ventricular anterior wall and the interventricular septum, (3) dilated systemic artery, (4) increased systolic excursion of the aortic or truncal valve cusps.[1-3] In most instances, these defects can be differentiated from one another and from other forms of cyanotic congenital heart disease by two-dimensional echocardiography.[4-8]

TETRALOGY OF FALLOT

In the parasternal and apical long-axis views in patients with tetralogy of Fallot, pulmonary atresia with a ventricular septal defect, and truncus arteriosus, the anterior aortic or truncal root is displaced anterior to the interventricular septum (Fig. 9-1).[4-8] The area of echocardiographic dropout between the anterior aortic root and septum represents a ventricular septal defect in the outlet or infundibular septum. Varying degrees of aortic override can be seen in patients with conotruncal defects. The echocardiographic appearance of aortic override can be falsely created by a transducer positioned too high on the pre-

149

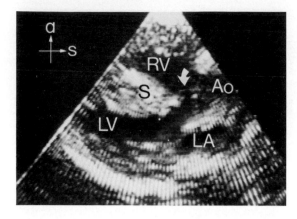

FIG. 9-1. *Parasternal long-axis view of a patient with tetralogy of Fallot. The dilated aorta (Ao) overrides the ventricular septum (S). An area of echocardiographic dropout representing a ventricular septal defect (arrow) is seen between the septum and anterior aortic root. The right ventricle (RV) and septum are thickened. a, anterior; LA, left atrium; LV, left ventricle; s, superior.*

cordium and can be obliterated by a transducer positioned too low on the precordium.[9] In the long-axis views, the systemic artery is usually dilated, and the systolic excursion of the semilunar valve cusps is increased.[8] Prominent hypertrophy of the right ventricular anterior wall and septum usually is present. From the long-axis views alone, it is not possible to distinguish tetralogy of Fallot from truncus arteriosus or pulmonary atresia with a ventricular septal defect.

   Patients with tetralogy of Fallot can be differentiated from patients with truncus arteriosus or pulmonary atresia with a ventricular septal defect by recording the pulmonary valve in the parasternal or subcostal short-axis views (Figs. 9-2 and 9-3). Care must be taken not to mistake the imperforate membrane in the right ventricular outflow tract in pulmonary atresia for a functioning pulmonary valve. Also, echoes arising from the left atrial appendage or a thickened and narrowed right ventricular infundibulum can mimic the pul-

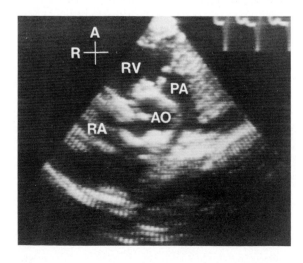

FIG. 9-2. *Parasternal short-axis view through the base of the heart from a patient with tetralogy of Fallot. The pulmonary valve is thickened and the valve annulus is narrowed. The main pulmonary artery (PA) and its branches are diminished in caliber. A, anterior; AO, aorta; R, right; RA, right atrium; RV, right ventricle.*

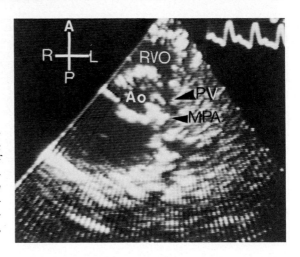

FIG. 9-3. *Parasternal short-axis view through the base of the heart from a patient with tetralogy of Fallot. The right ventricular outflow tract (RVO), pulmonary valve annulus (PV), and main pulmonary artery (MPA) are narrowed. A, anterior; Ao, aorta; L, left; P, posterior; R, right.*

monary valve in real time. To avoid these errors, the pulmonary valve opening and closure should be recorded by taking a simultaneous M-mode echocardiogram from the area in question on the two-dimensional echocardiogram.

In tetralogy of Fallot, right ventricular outflow obstruction can occur in the subvalvar, valvar, and/or supravalvar areas. In the short-axis views, the subvalvar area (infundibulum) is often hypertrophic and narrowed (Fig. 9-3).[6] The pulmonary valve is usually thickened and domed, and the pulmonary valve annulus is narrowed (Fig. 9-2). Stenosis of the right and left pulmonary artery branches can be detected in the short-axis and suprasternal notch views (Fig. 9-4). Absence of the left pulmonary artery, which is sometimes seen in patients with tetralogy of Fallot, can also be detected in the short-axis views (Fig. 9-5). Serial assessment of pulmonary artery size by two-dimensional echocardiography is a useful technique for determining the effect of surgical intervention on pulmonary blood flow in these patients. Since the parasternal short-axis view may not pass through the pulmonary arteries at their maximum diameter, pulmonary artery size can be underestimated in this view. In the suprasternal notch long-axis view, the right pulmonary artery is seen in cross section as it passes beneath the aortic arch. This view provides a reproducible plane in which to measure serially the maximum diameter of the right pulmonary artery at its origin from the main pulmonary artery. In addition, the suprasternal notch short-axis plane, which images the right pulmonary artery along its entire length, is especially useful for detecting peripheral stenosis of the right pulmonary artery. The left pulmonary artery, which passes out of the plane of the short-axis views just beyond its takeoff from the main pulmonary artery, is more difficult to evaluate by two-dimensional echocardiography. The suprasternal notch long-axis view can help detect stenosis of the left pulmonary artery (Fig. 9-4).

In a sweep from the base to the apex of the normal heart in the short-axis plane, the anterior aortic root is at the same level as the ventricular septum. In

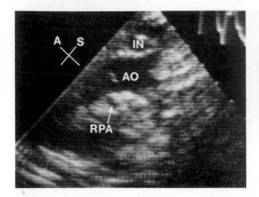
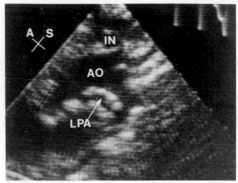

FIG. 9-4. *Suprasternal notch long-axis views through the right pulmonary artery (RPA) and left pulmonary artery (LPA) from a patient with tetralogy of Fallot. The branch pulmonary arteries are severely narrowed in this patient. A, anterior; AO, aorta; IN, innominate vein; S, superior.*

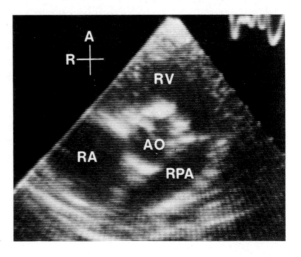

FIG. 9-5. *Parasternal short-axis view from a patient with tetralogy of Fallot following patch closure of the ventricular septal defect and pulmonary valvotomy. The left pulmonary artery is absent. Only the right pulmonary artery (RPA) arises from the main pulmonary artery. A, anterior; AO, aorta; R, right; RA, right atrium; RV, right ventricle.*

conotruncal defects with aortic override, the anterior aortic root is positioned anterior to the level of the septum in the short-axis sweep. The long- and short-axis views are also useful for evaluating the size of the ventricular septal defect and the presence of hypertrophic muscle bundles in the right ventricle (Fig. 9-6).

In the apical and subcostal four-chamber views in tetralogy of Fallot (Fig. 9-7), the right ventricle is thickened, dilated, and usually apex forming. Because of the decreased pulmonary blood flow, the left atrium is normal or decreased in size. Cranial angulation in the four-chamber views allows identifi-

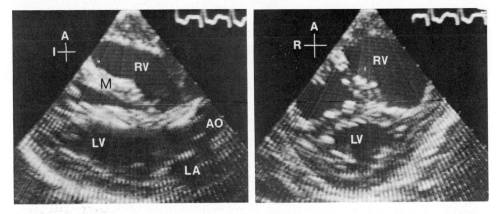

FIG. 9-6. *Parasternal long-(left) and short-(right) axis views from a patient who has undergone surgical repair of tetralogy of Fallot. The ventricular septal patch appears in place on the long-axis view. Residual hypertrophy of the right ventricle (RV) and a prominent, hypertrophic muscle bundle (M) are present. The RV is dilated because of residual tricuspid insufficiency. A, anterior; AO, aorta; I, inferior; LA, left atrium; LV, left ventricle; R, right.*

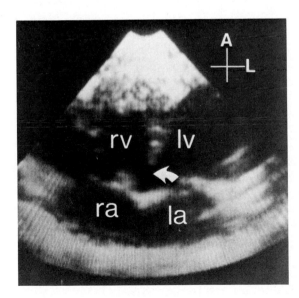

FIG. 9-7. *Apical four-chamber view from a patient with tetralogy of Fallot. The transducer is angled cranially in order to visualize the ventricular septal defect (arrow). The right ventricle (rv) is thickened and apex forming. A, apex; L, left; la, left atrium; lv, left ventricle; ra, right atrium.*

cation of the anterior ventricular septal defect and identification of the aorta arising above both ventricles.

Approximately 25 percent of patients with tetralogy of Fallot have a right-sided aortic arch that can be detected in the suprasternal notch long-axis view. In the suprasternal notch long-axis view in the normal left-sided aortic arch, the entire aortic arch can be imaged in a plane passing between the right nipple and left scapular tip. In patients with a right aortic arch, only portions of the aortic arch can be seen in the standard suprasternal notch long-axis view. The entire right aortic arch can be imaged in a plane passing between the right nipple and right scapular tip.

Tetralogy of Fallot Following Surgical Repair

In patients with tetralogy of Fallot who have undergone surgical repair, the ventricular septal defect patch can be seen positioned obliquely from the septum to the anteriorly displaced aortic root. In some patients, bright echoes can be seen arising from a patch across the right ventricular outflow tract. The parasternal and subcostal short-axis views can be used to detect aneurysmal dilatation of the infundibulum or outflow patch in the postoperative patient. The appearance of conduits will be discussed in Chapter 13.

Patients who have undergone repair of tetralogy of Fallot frequently have paradoxical septal motion. Paradoxical septal motion can be caused by right bundle branch block, the presence of a septal patch, or residual pulmonary or tricuspid insufficiency. Dilatation of the inferior vena cava, right atrium, and right ventricle with paradoxical septal motion should suggest the possibility of tricuspid insufficiency (Fig. 9-6). During a peripheral venous contrast injection in patients with tricuspid insufficiency, contrast echoes reflux into the inferior vena cava and hepatic veins during systole.[10] In diastole, reflux of contrast into the inferior vena cava and hepatic veins occurs normally during atrial contraction. In children with a rapid heart rate, a frame-by-frame analysis of the contrast injection is necessary to distinguish true systolic tricuspid insufficiency from normal diastolic reflux. The contrast injection can also be used to detect residual right-to-left shunting in postoperative patients.

Following pulmonary valvotomy or patching of the outflow tract, pulmonary insufficiency usually occurs. On the two-dimensional echocardiogram, pulmonary insufficiency causes right ventricular volume overload, paradoxical septal motion, and prominent pulsations in the main and branch pulmonary arteries. These pulsations are especially noticeable in the cross-sectional view of the right pulmonary artery from the suprasternal notch.

The detection of residual right ventricular outflow obstruction by two-dimensional echocardiography can be difficult, especially since right ventricular hypertrophy can persist for years even with a good surgical repair. In patients who have undergone surgical repair of tetralogy of Fallot, we can diagnose significant residual right ventricular outflow obstruction only when there is gross deformity and narrowing of the outflow tract in the short-axis views.

We have seen several patients who developed subaortic stenosis following surgical repair of tetralogy of Fallot. On the two-dimensional echocardiogram, these patients had left ventricular hypertrophy and narrowing of the left ventricular outflow tract caused by the oblique position of the septal patch or by a previously undetected fibromuscular shelf.

Congenital Absence of the Pulmonary Valve with Tetralogy of Fallot

On the M-mode and two-dimensional echocardiogram, patients with congenital absence of the pulmonary valve with tetralogy of Fallot have a dilated aorta overriding the ventricular septum, right ventricular dilatation and hypertrophy, and a narrowed right ventricular outflow tract.[11] In addition, signs of pulmonary insufficiency such as right ventricular volume overload, paradoxical septal motion, and prominent pulmonary artery pulsation are present. In the parasternal and subcostal short-axis views, the pulmonary annulus is narrowed and there is no evidence of pulmonary valve leaflets (Fig. 9-8). In the short-axis and suprasternal notch views, there is massive dilatation of the main and, especially, the right pulmonary arteries (Fig. 9-8 and 9-9).

PULMONARY ATRESIA WITH A VENTRICULAR SEPTAL DEFECT

In the long-axis and four-chamber views, there are no constant features that distinguish pulmonary atresia with a ventricular septal defect from tetralogy of Fallot or truncus arteriosus. Because of the large right-to-left ventricular shunt, patients with pulmonary atresia and a ventricular septal defect usually have a well-developed, dilated right ventricle. They also have a dilated aorta overriding the ventricular septum, a large subaortic ventricular septal defect, and right ventricular and septal thickening.

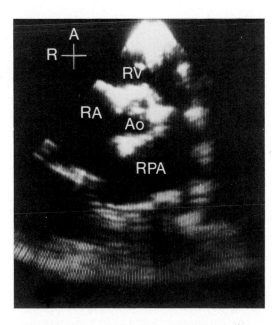

FIG. 9-8. *Parasternal short-axis view from a patient with congenital absence of the pulmonary valve and tetralogy of Fallot. The pulmonary valve annulus is narrowed, and the valve leaflets are absent. There is massive dilatation of the main and right pulmonary artery (RPA). A, anterior; Ao, aorta; R, right; RA, right atrium; RV, right ventricle.*

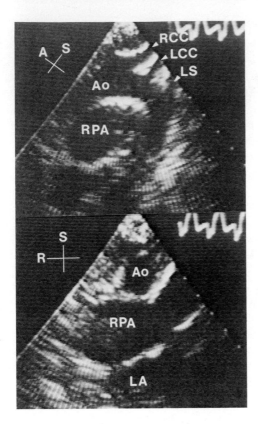

FIG. 9-9. *Suprasternal notch long-(**top**) and short-(**bottom**) axis views from a patient with congenital absence of the pulmonary valve and tetralogy of Fallot. The right pulmonary artery (RPA) is massively dilated. This degree of RPA dilatation is not commonly seen in other forms of congenital heart disease. A, anterior; Ao, aorta, LA, left atrium; LCC, left common carotid artery; LS, left subclavian artery; R, right; RCC, right common carotid artery; S, superior.*

In the parasternal and subcostal short-axis views in some cases, the right ventricular outflow tract seems to end blindly, and the main pulmonary artery and its branches cannot be imaged. Patients with these echocardiographic findings cannot be distinguished from patients with truncus arteriosus or severe tetralogy of Fallot. In the short-axis views in other cases, a small main pulmonary artery and bifurcation are imaged continuous with the right ventricular outflow tract but separated from it by a bright echo situated where a pulmonary valve would normally be (Fig. 9-10). This bright echo arises from an imperforate membrane and can resemble, at first glance, a small, dysplastic pulmonary valve. The imperforate membrane can be differentiated from a pulmonary valve by taking an M-mode echocardiogram from the two-dimensional echocardiogram. The M-mode echocardiogram of the imperforate membrane shows a thick line with a sine-wave motion and no evidence of a semilunar valve opening or closure. Peripheral venous contrast echocardiography in the short-axis views can also help distinguish an imperforate membrane from a dysplastic pulmonary valve. In tetralogy of Fallot with a functional pulmonary valve, contrast echoes flow forward from the right ventricle to the pulmonary artery. In patients with pulmonary atresia and a ventricular

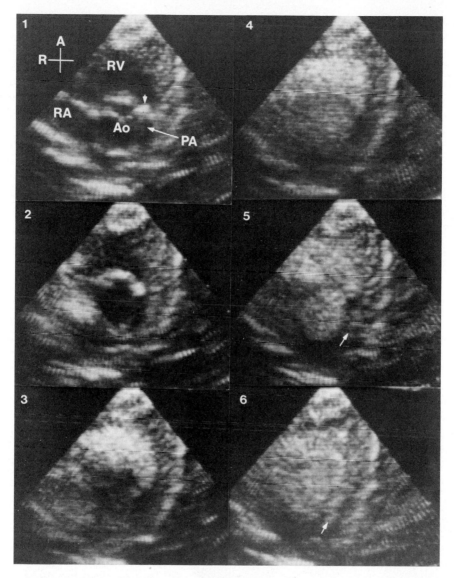

FIG. 9-10. *Peripheral venous contrast injection in the short-axis view in an infant with pulmonary atresia and a ventricular septal defect.* (**1**) *Prior to the contrast injection, an imperforate membrane (arrow) is seen in the area normally occupied by the pulmonary valve. The right ventricle (RV) is thickened and the aorta (Ao) is enlarged. The main pulmonary artery (PA) is small. A, anterior; R, right; RA, right atrium.* (**2** *and* **3**) *Contrast echoes are filling the right atrium and right ventricle. No contrast echoes have passed forward into the pulmonary artery.* (**4**) *The ascending aorta is filled with contrast echoes that arrive by way of a right-to-left ventricular shunt. The pulmonary artery is still free of contrast echoes.* (**5** *and* **6**) *Contrast echoes (arrows) are seen filling the pulmonary artery retrograde from bronchial collateral vessels arising from the descending aorta. The flow pattern shown by the contrast echocardiogram proves the diagnosis of pulmonary valve atresia.*

septal defect, contrast echoes fill the right atrium and right ventricle; however, contrast echoes do not flow forward from the right ventricle into the main pulmonary artery. Contrast echoes passing from right to left across the ventricular septal defect fill the left ventricle and ascending aorta. Following opacification of the ascending aorta, the main pulmonary artery fills retrograde with contrast echoes that arrive by way of a patent ductus arteriosus or bronchial collateral vessels. In order to detect the lack of forward flow across the imperforate membrane and the retrograde filling of the main pulmonary artery, the contrast echocardiogram must be reviewed carefully in slow motion.

In pulmonary atresia with a ventricular septal defect, the suprasternal notch views are useful for serial assessment of pulmonary artery size, especially in postoperative patients. It should be noted, however, that bronchial arteries cannot be distinguished with certainty from small pulmonary arteries in the suprasternal notch views.

PERSISTENT TRUNCUS ARTERIOSUS

In the parasternal and apical long-axis views, most patients with truncus arteriosus are indistinguishable from patients with tetralogy of Fallot or pulmonary atresia with a ventricular septal defect. A dilated truncal vessel overrides the ventricular septum. There is right ventricular and septal thickening and a large, subaortic ventricular septal defect (Fig. 9-11). In some cases, a few additional echocardiographic findings that suggest the diagnosis of truncus arteriosus may be present. If there is truncal valve insufficiency, left and right ventricular volume overload and paradoxical septal motion may be seen. In some cases of truncal valve insufficiency, a reverse doming of the truncal valve into the left ventricular outflow tract can be seen (Fig. 9-11). A few pa-

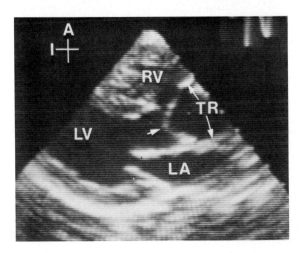

FIG. 9-11. *Parasternal long-axis view from a patient with persistent truncus arteriosus and truncal insufficiency. The dilated truncal vessel (TR) is overriding the ventricular septum. A large ventricular septal defect is present. The right ventricle (RV) and septum are thickened. The left ventricle (LV) is dilated because of truncal insufficiency. Reverse doming (arrow) of the truncal valve is seen. A, anterior; I, inferior; LA, left atrium.*

tients exhibit signs of truncal valve stenosis that are identical to the signs of aortic valve stenosis. In many instances, the left atrial dimensions will increase due to increased pulmonary blood flow—a rare finding in tetralogy and pulmonary atresia. Because of the large blood flow from the truncus into the pulmonary arteries in diastole, prominent pulsations are usually seen in the descending aorta in the subcostal views. Descending aortic pulsations are usually normal in patients with tetralogy or pulmonary atresia. Approximately 35 percent of patients with truncus arteriosus have a right-sided aortic arch detectable by suprasternal notch echocardiography.

In the parasternal or subcostal short-axis views, the finding of a systemic artery with four semilunar valve cusps should suggest the diagnosis of truncus arteriosus (Fig. 9-12). Most patients with tetralogy of Fallot or pulmonary atresia have three aortic valve cusps while approximately 25 percent of patients with truncus arteriosus have four semilunar cusps.[12]

When the pulmonary arteries are seen arising directly from the ascending aorta, the diagnosis of truncus arteriosus can be made with certainty. In some instances, the pulmonary arteries can be seen in the long-axis views arising from the posterior aspect of the ascending aorta (Fig. 9-13). Also, the pulmonary arteries can be seen arising from the left lateral or posterior aspect of the ascending truncal vessel in the parasternal and subcostal short-axis views (Figs. 9-14 and 9-15). If both pulmonary artery branches arise from a common site, a type I or II truncus arteriosus is present. It may be difficult to determine whether the pulmonary artery branches arise from the truncus by way of a short main pulmonary artery segment (type I) or by way of separate side-by-side ostia (type II). The diagnosis of truncus arteriosus can also be made by imaging the origin of the pulmonary arteries from the ascending aorta in the suprasternal notch views (Figs. 9-16 and 9-17). By tilting the transducer from right to left in these views, it occasionally is possible to follow a main pulmo-

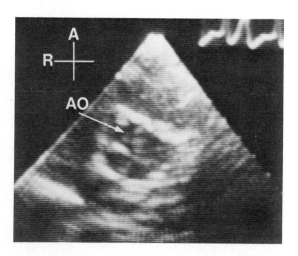

FIG. 9-12. *Parasternal short-axis view from a patient with truncus arteriosus. The aortic or truncal valve has four cusps. A, anterior; AO, aorta; R, right.*

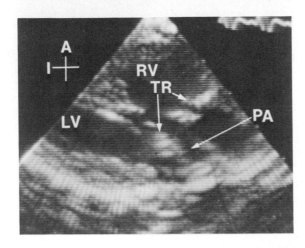

FIG. 9-13. *Parasternal long-axis view from a patient with truncus arteriosus. The truncal vessel (TR) is dilated and overrides the ventricular septum. A large ventricular septal defect is seen. The main pulmonary artery segment (PA) arises from the posterior aspect of the truncus. A, anterior; I, inferior; LV, left ventricle; RV, right ventricle.*

nary artery segment to its bifurcation into right and left branches (type I truncus). In other cases, only a single pulmonary artery can be seen arising from the ascending aorta (type III truncus, Fig. 9-17).

DOUBLE OUTLET RIGHT VENTRICLE

In patients with double outlet right ventricle, both great arteries arise primarily from the right ventricle. The exit of blood from the left ventricle is by way of a ventricular septal defect that can be committed to either the aorta, the pulmonary artery, both, or neither. Double outlet right ventricle can occur with or without pulmonary stenosis. Usually, the great vessels are situated side by side with the aorta on the right; however, the great vessels can be po-

FIG. 9-14. *Parasternal short-axis view from a patient with type I truncus arteriosus. A short main pulmonary artery segment (PA) and the two pulmonary artery branches are seen arising from the posterior aspect of the truncus (TR). The echocardiographic dropout between the right ventricle (RV) and truncus represents a ventricular septal defect. A, anterior; LA; left atrium; R, right; RA, right atrium.*

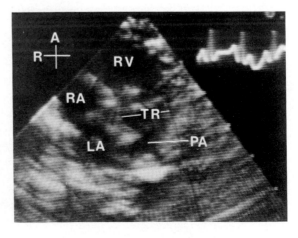

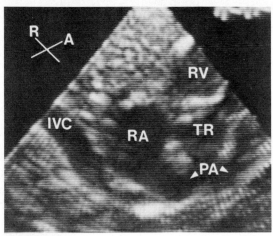

FIG. 9-15. *Subcostal short-axis view from a patient with type I truncus arteriosus. The common pulmonary artery segment (PA) is seen arising from the posterior aspect of the truncus (TR) and bifurcating into the two pulmonary artery branches (arrows). A, anterior; IVC, inferior vena cava; R, right; RA, right atrium; RV, right ventricle.*

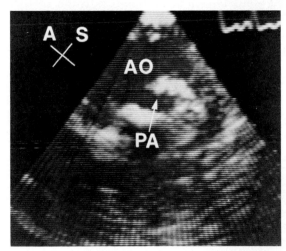

FIG. 9-16. *Suprasternal notch long-axis view from a patient with type I truncus arteriosus. The main pulmonary artery (PA) is seen arising from the posterior aspect of the ascending aorta (AO). The pulmonary artery branches could be imaged by tilting the transducer from right to left. A, anterior; S, superior.*

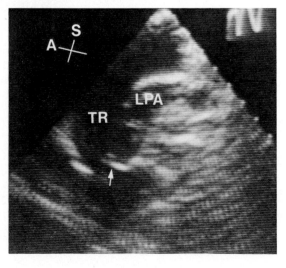

FIG. 9-17. *Suprasternal notch long-axis view from a patient with type III truncus arteriosus. The left pulmonary artery (LPA) arose from the posterior aspect of the ascending truncus (TR). The right pulmonary artery, which arose from the transverse arch, could not be imaged in this view. The truncal valve can also be seen (arrow). A, anterior; S, superior.*

sitioned normally or can be d- or l-transposed. The subaortic conus persists to a varying degree and intervenes between the aortic and mitral valves (mitral–aortic discontinuity). The aortic valve is, therefore, located more superiorly than usual. Double outlet right ventricle can occur with transposition of the great arteries and a subpulmonary ventricular septal defect (Taussig–Bing malformation). In this abnormality, there is levoposition of the pulmonary conus so that the pulmonary artery spatially overrides the left ventricle. The subpulmonic conus persists to a varying degree and intervenes between the pulmonary and mitral valves (mitral–pulmonary discontinuity).[12]

In the parasternal long-axis view in patients with double outlet right ventricle, the aorta usually arises entirely from the right ventricle (Fig. 9-18). Depending on the spatial relations of the aorta and pulmonary artery, one or both great arteries can be seen in the long-axis view arising from the right ventricle. In patients with double outlet right ventricle and transposition of the great arteries, the two great vessels arise from the right ventricle in a parallel orientation with the posterior pulmonary artery partially overriding the ventricular septum (Fig. 9-19). In this situation, the posterior great vessel can be identified as the pulmonary artery by its sharp posterior angulation toward the lungs in the long-axis view.[8] The persistence of the subaortic or subpulmonic conus is visualized in the long-axis views as an increased distance (in the inferior–superior direction) between the anterior mitral valve leaflet and the semilunar valve.

In the normal heart, the right ventricular outflow tract and pulmonary artery wrap around the aorta and create a "circle-sausage" appearance in the short-axis views. In double outlet right ventricle, the great vessels usually arise in a parallel fashion from the right ventricle and appear as "double circles" in the short-axis view through the base of the heart.[7,13] In the most usual form of double outlet right ventricle, the great arteries are side by side with the aorta to the right of the pulmonary artery (Fig. 9-20). In other patients, the aorta can be seen to the right and anterior of the pulmonary artery, directly anterior to the pulmonary artery, or to the left and anterior of the pulmonary

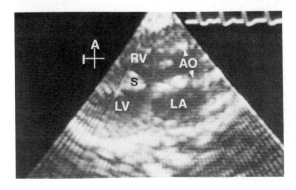

FIG. 9-18. *Parasternal long-axis view from a patient with double outlet right ventricle. The aorta (AO) arises entirely from the right ventricle (RV). There is an increased distance between the mitral and aortic valves due to persistence of the subaortic conus. The pulmonary artery could not be seen in this view. A, anterior; I, inferior; LA, left atrium; LV, left ventricle; S, septum.*

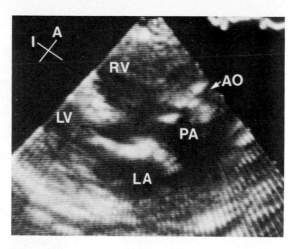

FIG. 9-19. *Parasternal long-axis view from a patient with double outlet right ventricle and transposition of the great arteries. Both great vessels arise from the right ventricle (RV) in a parallel fashion with the posterior pulmonary artery (PA) partially overriding the ventricular septum. Persistence of the subpulmonic conus causes the wide separation between the mitral and pulmonic valves. A, anterior; AO, aorta; I, inferior; LA, left atrium; LV, left ventricle.*

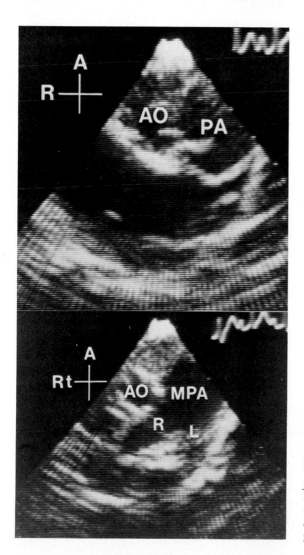

FIG. 9-20. *Parasternal short-axis views from a patient with double outlet right ventricle and side-by-side great arteries. With cranial angulation of the transducer, the vessel on the left can be seen to bifurcate into right (R) and left (L) branches, thus distinguishing it as the pulmonary artery (MPA). A, anterior; AO, aorta; Rt, right; PA, pulmonary artery.*

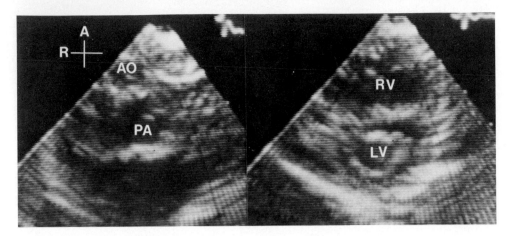

FIG. 9-21. *Short-axis sweep from the base* (**left**) *to the apex* (**right**) *of the heart from a patient with double outlet right ventricle* (*RV*) *and d-transposition of the great arteries. The aorta* (*AO*) *is anterior and to the right of the pulmonary artery* (*PA*). *Both great vessels arise primarily from the right ventricle above the level of the ventricular septum; however, the pulmonary artery partially overrides the septum. A, anterior; LV, left ventricle; R, right.*

artery. In the short-axis view, the pulmonary artery can be distinguished from the aorta by angulating the transducer superiorly to see which vessel bifurcates into pulmonary artery branches. In double outlet right ventricle with pulmonary stenosis, a thickened, domed pulmonary valve and a narrowed pulmonary valve annulus frequently can be seen in the short-axis views. In a sweep in the short-axis view from the base to the apex of the heart, both great arteries are positioned anterior to the level of the ventricular septum. In a short-axis sweep in patients with double outlet right ventricle and transposition, the posterior pulmonary artery partially overrides the ventricular septum (Fig. 9-21).

Because of the anatomic variations found in patients with double outlet right ventricle, it is not always possible to distinguish double outlet right ventricle with normally related great arteries from severe tetralogy of Fallot by two-dimensional echocardiography. On the other hand, it is not always possible to distinguish double outlet right ventricle with transposition of the great arteries from d-transposition of the great arteries with a ventricular septal defect and overriding pulmonary artery.

REFERENCES

1. Chung KJ, Alexson CG, Manning JA, Gramiak R: Echocardiography in truncus arteriosus: The value of pulmonic valve detection. Circulation 48: 281, 1973

2. Morris DC, Felner JM, Schlant RC, Franch RH: Echocardiographic diagnosis of tetralogy of Fallot. Am J Cardiol 36: 908, 1975
3. Assad-Morell JL, Seward JB, Tajik AJ, Hagler DJ, Giuliani ER, Ritter DG: Echophonocardiographic and contrast studies in conditions associated with systemic arterial trunk overriding the ventricular septum: Truncus arteriosus, tetralogy of Fallot, and pulmonary atresia with ventricular septal defect. Circulation 53: 663, 1976
4. Sahn DJ, Terry R, O'Rourke R, Leopold G, Friedman WF: Multiple crystal cross-sectional echocardiography in the diagnosis of cyanotic congenital heart disease. Circulation 50: 230, 1974
5. Henry WL, Maron BJ, Griffith JM, Redwood DR, Epstein SE: Differential diagnosis of anomalies of the great arteries by real-time two-dimensional echocardiography. Circulation 51: 283, 1975
6. Caldwell RL, Weyman AE, Hurwitz RA, Girod DA, Feigenbaum H: Right ventricular outflow tract assessment by cross-sectional echocardiography in tetralogy of Fallot. Circulation 59: 395, 1979
7. DiSessa TG, Hagan AD, Pope C, Samtoy L, Friedman WF: Two-dimensional echocardiographic characteristics of double outlet right ventricle. Am J Cardiol 44: 1146, 1979
8. Hagler DJ, Tajik AJ, Seward JB, Mair DD, Ritter DG: Wide-angle two-dimensional echocardiographic profiles of conotruncal abnormalities. Mayo Clin Proc 55: 73, 1980
9. French JW, Popp R: Variability of echocardiographic discontinuity in double outlet right ventricle and truncus arteriosus. Circulation 51: 848, 1975
10. Lieppe W, Behar VS, Scallion R, Kisslo JA: Detection of tricuspid regurgitation with two-dimensional echocardiography and peripheral vein injections. Circulation 57: 128, 1978
11. Nagai Y, Komatsu Y, Nakamura K, Sato Y, Takao A: Echocardiographic findings of congenital absence of the pulmonary valve with tetralogy of Fallot. Chest 75: 481, 1979
12. Goor DA, Lillehei CW: Congenital Malformations of the Heart. New York, Grune and Stratton, 1975
13. Henry WL, Maron BJ, Griffith JM: Cross-sectional echocardiography in the diagnosis of congenital heart disease: Identification of the relation of the ventricles and great arteries. Circulation 56: 267, 1977

CHAPTER 10

Transposition of the Great Arteries

ECHOCARDIOGRAPHIC DIAGNOSIS OF TRANSPOSITION

In this chapter, we will discuss d- and l-transposition of the great arteries in situs solitus. The term transposition describes the situation where the aorta arises from the anatomic right ventricle and the pulmonary artery arises from the anatomic left ventricle. The aorta is usually anterior to the pulmonary artery. The term d-transposition or simple transposition of the great arteries will be used to describe the situation where the anatomic right ventricle is located to the right of the anatomic left ventricle. The term l-transposition or l-transposition with ventricular inversion will be used to describe the situation where the anatomic right ventricle is to the left of the anatomic left ventricle.

Before making the two-dimensional echocardiographic diagnosis of d- or l-transposition, it is necessary: (1) to define the spatial relations of the great vessels, (2) to image the bifurcation of the posterior pulmonary artery, (3) to determine the atrioventricular connections.

Spatial Relations of the Great Vessels

In the normal parasternal short-axis view at the base of the heart, the aorta is seen in cross section as a posterior circular structure. The right ventricular outflow tract courses from right to left anterior to the aorta and reaches the pulmonary valve to the left of the aortic valve. The appearance of the normal great vessels in the short-axis view has been called the "circle-sausage" appearance.[1] In d- and l-transposition, the great arteries exit from the heart in a parallel fashion. Both great arteries are seen in cross section in the short-axis views and appear as "double circles."[1,2] In d-transposition, the anterior aorta is usually to the right of the posterior pulmonary artery (Fig. 10-1). In l-transposition with ventricular inversion, the aorta lies anterior and to the left of the pulmonary artery (Fig. 10-2). In order to image both semilunar valves in d-transposition, the parasternal short-axis plane may have to be oriented more horizontally than usual.[1]

Frequently in transposition complexes, the vessels do not have a left–right relationship, and the aorta lies immediately anterior to the pulmonary artery (Fig. 10-3). Also, in d-transposition of the great vessels, the aorta can be situated to the left of the pulmonary artery and still arise from an anatomic

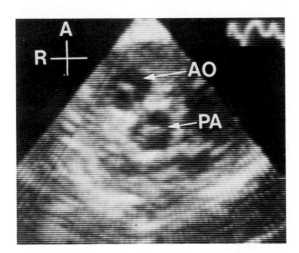

FIG. 10-1. *Parasternal short-axis view from a patient with d-transposition of the great arteries. Because of their parallel exit from the heart, the great vessels are seen in cross section in the short-axis view as "double circles." The aorta (AO) is anterior and to the right of the pulmonary artery (PA). Both semilunar valves are tricuspid. A, anterior; R, right.*

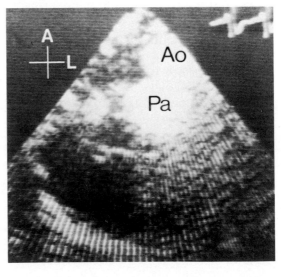

FIG. 10-2. *Contrast injection in the parasternal short-axis view from a patient with l-transposition and a right-to-left ventricular shunt. The great vessels are seen in cross section as "double circles." The aorta (Ao) is anterior and to the left of the pulmonary artery (Pa). A, anterior; L, left.*

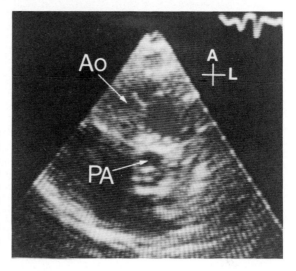

FIG. 10-3. *Parasternal short-axis view through the base of the heart from a patient with d-transposition and pulmonary stenosis. The aorta (Ao) is positioned directly anterior to the pulmonary artery (PA). The pulmonary valve is bicuspid, and the pulmonary valve annulus is narrowed. A, anterior; L, left.*

right ventricle located to the right of the anatomic left ventricle (Fig. 10-4). Similarly, in l-transposition, a variety of left–right positions of the great vessels can occur. The spatial relationship of the aorta and pulmonary artery in the short-axis views allows the detection of transposition of the great vessels but does not always allow differentiation of simple d-transposition of the great arteries from l-transposition with ventricular inversion. For this differentiation to be made, the atrioventricular connections must be determined.

The parallel exit of the great vessels from the ventricles can be imaged in the parasternal and apical long-axis planes (Fig. 10-5 and 10-6).[3] The anterior aortic valve is usually superior to the posterior pulmonary valve. The posterior pulmonary artery has a sharp posterior angulation as it courses toward the lungs, in contrast to the normal heart where the posterior aorta lacks this sharp

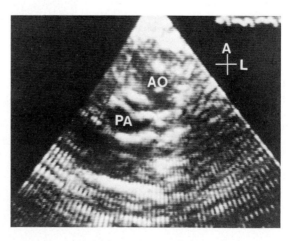

FIG. 10-4. *Parasternal short-axis view from a patient with d-transposition of the great vessels. In this patient, the aorta (AO) is anterior and to the left of the pulmonary artery (PA). The diagnosis of d-transposition was based on imaging the anatomic right ventricle to the right of the anatomic left ventricle in the four-chamber views. A, anterior; L, left.*

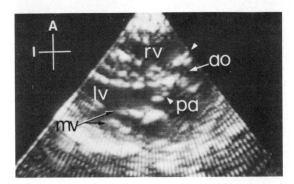

FIG. 10-5. *Parasternal long-axis view from a patient with d-transposition. Because of the parallel exit of the great arteries from the heart, both great vessels are seen simultaneously in the long-axis view. The anterior aorta (ao) is seen arising from the right ventricle (rv), and the posterior pulmonary artery (pa) is seen arising from the left ventricle (lv). Note the posterior sweep of the pulmonary artery toward the lungs. Arrows indicate the semilunar valves. The aortic valve is superior to the pulmonary valve. A, anterior; I, inferior; mv, mitral valve.*

FIG. 10-6. *Parasternal long-axis view from a patient with d-transposition. Note the parallel exit of the great vessels from the heart and the sharp posterior sweep of the posterior pulmonary artery (pa). Arrows indicate the semilunar valves. a, anterior; ao, aorta; i, inferior; la, left atrium; lv, left ventricle; rv, right ventricle.*

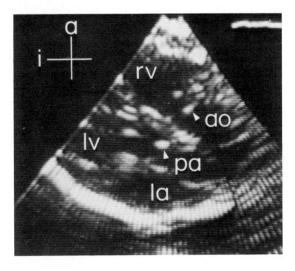

posterior angulation as it exits from the heart. Occasionally, it is possible to image a large part of the aortic arch arising from the anterior right ventricle (Fig. 10-7).

The Bifurcation of the Pulmonary Artery

Unusual transducer positions high on the precordium and unusual cardiac orientation can create the appearance of "double circles" in the short-axis views. In order to prove that the posterior circle is the pulmonary artery, the bifurcation of this vessel into two pulmonary artery branches should be imaged.[4] The

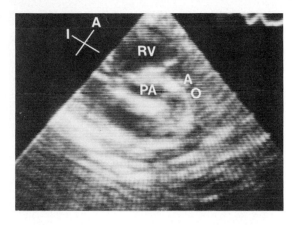

FIG. 10-7. *Parasternal long-axis view through the right ventricle (RV) from a patient with d-transposition. The entire aortic arch (AO) can be seen arising from the anterior right ventricle (RV). A, anterior; I, inferior; PA, pulmonary artery.*

pulmonary artery bifurcation can be imaged by tilting the transducer cranially in the short-axis planes (Fig. 10-8). The vessel that bifurcates into two branches is the pulmonary artery. The pulmonary artery bifurcation can also be imaged in the subcostal short-axis and four-chamber views (Fig. 10-9).[5]

The Atrioventricular Connections

In transposition complexes, the spatial relationships of the two great vessels is variable; therefore, the distinction between d- and l-transposition depends on locating the anatomic right ventricle. In the apical and subcostal four-chamber views, the anatomic right ventricle has an atrioventricular valve situated closer to the cardiac apex and has a moderator band. In d-transposition in situs solitus, the anatomic right ventricle is located to the right of the anatomic left ventricle and connects to the right atrium (Fig. 10-10). In l-transposition in

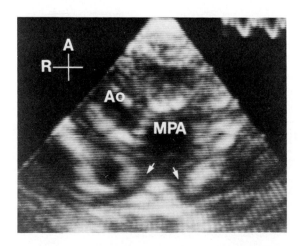

FIG. 10-8. *Parasternal short-axis view from a patient with d-transposition. The aorta (Ao) is to the right and anterior of the pulmonary artery (MPA). The transducer has been directed superiorly in order to image the pulmonary artery bifurcation (arrows). Imaging of the bifurcation proves that the posterior vessel is the pulmonary artery. A, anterior; R, right.*

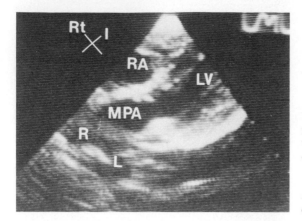

FIG. 10-9. *Subcostal view from a patient with d-transposition. The main pulmonary artery (MPA) is seen arising from the left ventricle (LV) and bifurcating into the right (R) and left (L) pulmonary artery branches. I, inferior; RA, right atrium; Rt, right.*

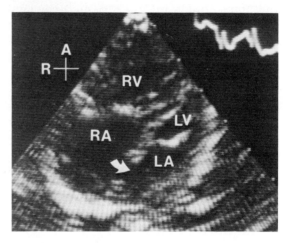

FIG. 10-10. *Apical four-chamber view from a patient with d-transposition following balloon atrial septostomy. A large atrial septal tear (arrow) is present. The right atrium (RA) and right ventricle (RV) are much larger than the left atrium (LA) and left ventricle (LV). A, apex; R, right.*

situs solitus, the anatomic right ventricle is located to the left of the anatomic left ventricle and connects to the left atrium (Fig. 10-11). The echocardiographic determinants of the atrioventricular connections in situs inversus and situs ambiguus will be discussed in detail in Chapter 14.

d-TRANSPOSITION OF THE GREAT ARTERIES

Chamber Sizes

In the apical and subcostal four-chamber views of patients with simple transposition of the great arteries, the right ventricle is thickened, enlarged, and apex forming. Usually, the right atrium and right ventricle are considerably

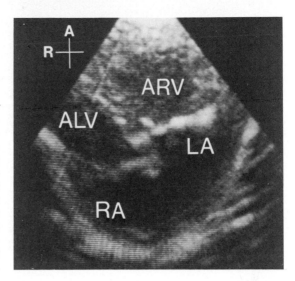

FIG. 10-11. *Apical four-chamber view from a patient with l-transposition and ventricular inversion. The left-sided atrioventricular valve is closer to the cardiac apex than the right-sided atrioventricular valve, indicating that the left atrioventricular valve is the tricuspid valve and that the anatomic right ventricle (ARV) is to the left of the anatomic left ventricle (ALV). A, apex; LA, left atrium; R, right; RA, right atrium.*

larger than the left atrium and left ventricle in the parasternal and apical planes.[6] The finding of an enlarged left ventricle on the two-dimensional echocardiogram suggests the presence of either pulmonic stenosis, patent ductus arteriosus, a ventricular septal defect, or persistent pulmonary artery hypertension.

In the short-axis views in most patients with simple transposition of the great arteries, the right ventricle is the dominant circular ventricle and the left ventricle is crescent shaped. The ventricular septal motion is usually flattened or frankly paradoxical. However, variations in the shapes of the two ventricles may relate to altered pressures exerted on both sides of the ventricular septum.

Associated Defects

Left ventricular outflow obstruction in d-transposition can occur at the valvar or subvalvar regions of the outflow tract. Valvar pulmonic stenosis in d-transposition is often associated with a bicuspid pulmonary valve. In these patients in the parasternal and subcostal short-axis views, the pulmonary valve has two cusps and the pulmonary valve annulus is often smaller than the aortic valve annulus (Fig. 10-3).

Subpulmonary stenosis in d-transposition can be due to a dynamic or fixed anatomic obstruction in the left ventricular outflow tract.[7,8] Dynamic left ventricular outflow obstruction is usually caused by the posterior displacement of the ventricular septum into the left ventricular outflow tract. Fixed anatomic subpulmonary stenosis is usually caused by a subpulmonary membrane or a fibromuscular shelf present in the left ventricular outflow tract. The parasternal and apical long-axis views are especially useful for detecting subpulmonary narrowing (Fig. 10-12).

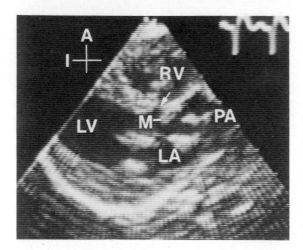

FIG. 10-12. *Parasternal long-axis view from a patient with d-transposition, a large ventricular septal defect (arrow), a subpulmonary membrane (M), and pulmonary valve stenosis. Note the thickened pulmonary valve and poststenotic dilatation of the pulmonary artery (PA). The left ventricle (LV) is thickened and dilated. A, anterior; I, inferior; LA, left atrium; RV, right ventricle.*

Ventricular septal defects associated with d-transposition usually occur in the membranous region of the ventricular septum (Fig. 10-12) but can also occur in the muscular and outlet ventricular septum. With a large ventricular septal defect and increased pulmonary blood flow, the left atrium and left ventricle can be enlarged.

d-Transposition After Balloon Atrial Septostomy

Balloon atrial septostomy can be performed using the two-dimensional echocardiogram to locate the position of the balloon catheter.[9] This technique is especially valuable for locating the balloon in the left atrium when only single plane angiographic equipment is available (Fig. 10-13).

After balloon atrial septostomy, the size of the atrial tear can be assessed using the two-dimensional echocardiogram. For this purpose, a combination of parasternal, apical, and subcostal views should be used (Fig. 10-10). When the tear is adequate, the torn edges of the atrial septum have a rapid, flicking motion within the atrium on the real-time recordings. In those patients who appear to have a large atrial septal tear with an unsatisfactory increase in the arterial oxygen content, two-dimensional contrast echocardiography can be used to determine the adequacy of the intra-atrial mixing. In a peripheral venous contrast injection in the apical four-chamber view, the amount of contrast echoes passing from right to left at atrial level is a rough indication of the degree of intra-atrial mixing.[9]

d-TRANSPOSITION AFTER INTRA-ATRIAL BAFFLE OPERATIONS

Several reports have described the M-mode echocardiographic appearance of the intra-atrial baffle in patients with d-transposition after the Mustard proce-

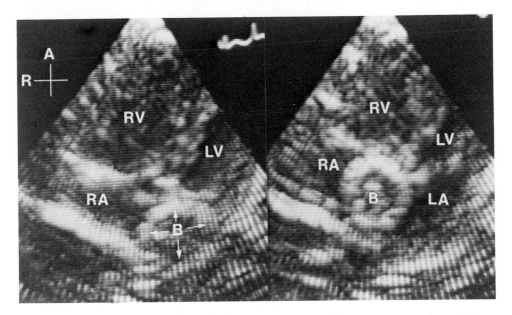

FIG. 10-13. *Apical four-chamber view of a balloon atrial septostomy performed in an infant with d-transposition.* **Left.** *The balloon (B) is inflated in the left atrium (LA). The right atrium (RA) and right ventricle (RV) are enlarged.* **Right.** *The balloon has been pulled across the atrial septum into the right atrium. A, apex; LV, left ventricle; R, right.*

dure.[10-12] The M-mode echocardiogram has been used to determine wall thicknesses and chamber dimensions in patients who have undergone the Mustard procedure. In those patients without significant postoperative defects, the right ventricular dimensions are considerably larger than the left ventricular dimensions. Also, the right ventricular anterior wall thickness is much greater than the left ventricular posterior wall thickness. On the M-mode echocardiogram, the findings of a dilated left ventricular cavity or a thickened left ventricular posterior wall suggest significant residual defects, such as subpulmonary stenosis, a ventricular septal defect, or pulmonary artery hypertension possibly related to pulmonary venous obstruction. The two-dimensional echocardiogram is especially useful for evaluating residual defects in patients who have undergone the Mustard operation.

The Course of the Baffle

The intra-atrial baffle divides the previous right and left atria into systemic and pulmonary venous atria. The baffle can be thought of as a conduit running between the superior and inferior venae cavae and the mitral valve. The systemic venous drainage passes under the conduit while the pulmonary venous drainage cascades over the conduit to reach the tricuspid valve. The systemic and pulmonary venous atria cannot be seen in their entirety in any one echocardiographic plane. Therefore, a combination of echocardiographic views is necessary for complete evaluation of all portions of the systemic and pulmonary venous atria. Peripheral venous contrast echocardiography has been especially useful in identifying the systemic venous atrium in each view. In the patients we have examined, the intra-atrial baffle was constructed from pericardium and had a phasic motion similar to the mitral valve. The phasic motion of the baffle may relate to changes in atrial volumes caused by respiration, and the amount of baffle motion is largely dependent upon the redundancy of the material used to construct the baffle.

In the parasternal and apical long-axis views, the intraatrial baffle stretches obliquely across the atrium with extensions anterosuperiorly and posteroinferiorly (Figs. 10-14 and 10-15). Anterior and inferior to the baffle, the midportion of the systemic venous atrium is seen communicating with the mitral valve and left ventricle. The superior vena caval and inferior vena caval portions of the sytemic venous atrium cannot be imaged in the long-axis views. Posterior and superior to the baffle, a portion of the pulmonary venous atrium can be seen. The pulmonary veins and the connection of the pulmonary venous atrium to the tricuspid valve cannot be seen in the long-axis views.

In the parasternal short-axis view, the upper portion of the systemic venous atrium courses from the area of the superior vena cava on the right toward the mitral valve on the left (Fig. 10-16). In addition, a portion of the pulmonary venous atrium can be seen posterior to the intra-atrial baffle.

In the apical four-chamber view, the systemic venous atrium between the inferior vena cava and the mitral valve can be imaged (Fig. 10-17). In this view, echoes arise from the anterior and posterior portions of the pericardial tube. With cranial angulation in the apical four-chamber view, the pulmonary venous atrium between the pulmonary veins and the tricuspid valve can be seen (Fig. 10-17). In this view, the pulmonary venous atrium is divided by the

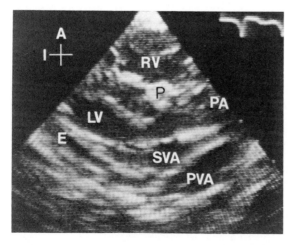

FIG. 10-14. *Parasternal long-axis view from a patient following the Mustard operation and patch (P) closure of a ventricular septal defect. The baffle is seen stretching across the atrium. Anterior and inferior to the baffle, the systemic venous atrium (SVA) is seen communicating with the mitral valve and left ventricle (LV). Posterior and superior to the baffle, a small portion of the pulmonary venous atrium (PVA) is seen. A small, posterior pericardial effusion (E) is present. A, anterior; I, inferior; PA, pulmonary artery; RV, right ventricle.*

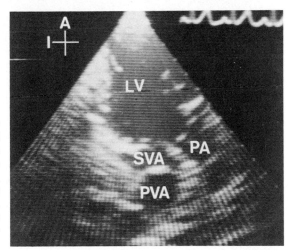

FIG. 10-15. *Apical long-axis view from a patient after the Mustard operation. The systemic venous atrium (SVA) is seen communicating with the left ventricle (LV). A portion of the pulmonary venous atrium (PVA) can be visualized. Note the posterior sweep of the pulmonary artery (PA). A, anterior; I, inferior.*

sharp angulation of the baffle into two portions—a portion receiving the pulmonary veins and a portion communicating with the tricuspid valve. With cranial angulation in the apical four-chamber view (Fig. 10-17, bottom), only the midportion of the systemic venous atrium can be imaged.

In the subcostal long-axis views, the junction of the inferior vena cava and the systemic venous atrium can be seen (Fig. 10-18). In some instances, the entire systemic venous atrium between the inferior vena cava and mitral valve can be imaged in the subcostal long-axis view. Frequently, the baffle and a portion of the pulmonary venous atrium are present in this view.

With cranial angulation, the junction between the superior vena cava and the systemic venous atrium and a part of the lower portion of the systemic venous atrium can be examined from the subcostal long-axis views (Fig. 10-19). The pulmonary venous atrium adjacent to the tricuspid valve is present in this view.

Baffle Leaks

During peripheral venous contrast injections in patients with baffle leaks, contrast echoes pass from the systemic venous atrium into the pulmonary venous atrium (Fig. 10-20). Contrast echocardiography is a highly sensitive technique for detecting baffle leaks that occur in approximately 90 percent of patients following the Mustard procedure. In many patients, right-to-left baffle leaks can be detected by contrast echocardiography even when the arterial oxygen saturation is normal.

Systemic and Pulmonary Venous Obstruction

Superior vena caval obstruction following the Mustard procedure is a relatively frequent complication. Angiographic flow patterns have been described

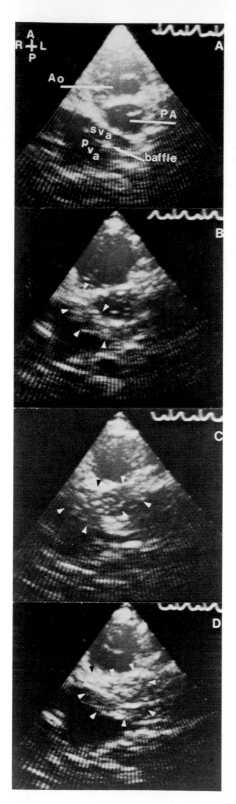

FIG. 10-16. **A.** *Parasternal short-axis view through the base of the heart in a patient with d-transposition following the Mustard operation. Because of the parallel exit of the great vessels from the heart, the aorta (Ao) and pulmonary artery (PA) are seen in cross section as "double circles." The aorta is anterior and to the right of the pulmonary artery. A superior portion of the systemic venous atrium (sva) can be seen anterior to the baffle. A portion of the pulmonary venous atrium (pva) can also be seen. A, anterior; L, left; P, posterior; R, right.* **B.** *Following a contrast injection into an arm vein, contrast echoes (arrows) are seen flowing in the superior portion of the systemic venous atrium toward the mitral valve.* **C** *and* **D.** *Contrast echoes (arrows) have filled the systemic venous atrium and reached the pulmonary artery.*

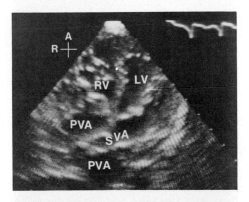

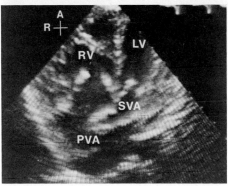

FIG. 10-17. Top. *Apical four-chamber view from a patient after the Mustard operation. The systemic venous atrium (SVA) between the inferior vena cava and the mitral valve can be seen. Echoes arise from the anterior and posterior walls of the baffle conduit. Portions of the pulmonary venous atrium (PVA) can be seen. Note the hypertrophy of the right ventricle (RV). A, apex; LV, left ventricle; R, right. Bottom. With cranial angulation from the standard four-chamber view, the entire pulmonary venous atrium (PVA) can be seen. The sharp angulation of the baffle divides the pulmonary venous atrium into two portions—a portion receiving the pulmonary veins and a portion communicating with the tricuspid valve and right ventricle (RV). The midportion of the systemic venous atrium (SVA) that communicates with the mitral valve and left ventricle (LV) can also be seen. A, apex; R, right.*

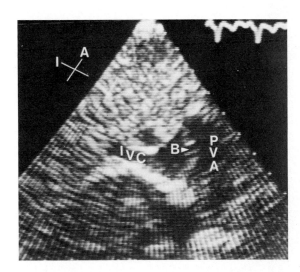

FIG. 10-18. *Subcostal long-axis view from a patient after the Mustard procedure. The junction of the inferior vena cava (IVC) and systemic venous atrium can be seen. A portion of the baffle (B) and a portion of the pulmonary venous atrium (PVA) can also be seen. A, anterior; I, inferior.*

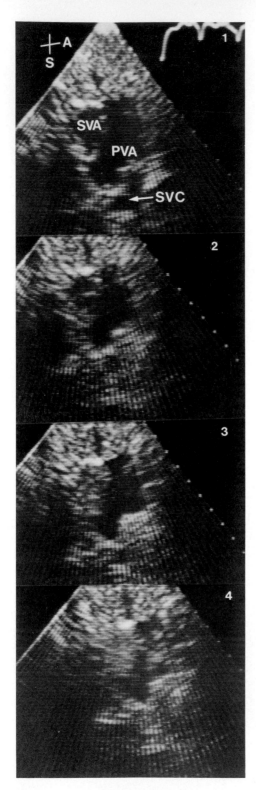

FIG. 10-19. 1. *Subcostal view from a patient after the Mustard operation. The junction of the superior vena cava (SVC) and systemic venous atrium and a part of the lower portion of the systemic venous atrium (SVA) can be seen. The pulmonary venous atrium (PVA) adjacent to the tricuspid valve can also be imaged. A, anterior; S, superior.* **2.** *Following a contrast injection into an arm vein, contrast echoes fill the junction of the superior vena cava and systemic venous atrium.* **3.** *Contrast echoes are seen in the lower portion of the systemic venous atrium.* **4.** *Because of a right-to-left baffle leak, contrast echoes are seen in the pulmonary venous atrium.*

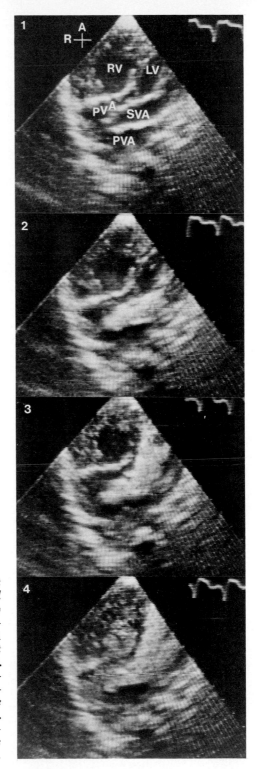

FIG. 10-20. *Peripheral venous contrast injection in a patient after the Mustard operation. 1. Apical four-chamber view prior to the contrast injection. The systemic and pulmonary venous atria (SVA and PVA) can be seen. A, apex; LV, left ventricle; R, right; RV, right ventricle. 2. Following an arm vein injection, the systemic venous atrium is filled with contrast echoes. 3. Contrast echoes have passed forward into the left ventricle. 4. Contrast echoes are seen in the pulmonary venous atrium and right ventricle because of a large right-to-left baffle leak.*

to diagnose complete, partial, and no superior vena caval obstruction.[13] At angiography in patients with no superior vena caval obstruction, an injection of
radiographic contrast material into the superior vena cava fills the systemic
venous atrium entirely from above. In patients with complete superior vena
caval obstruction, the radiographic contrast material injected into the superior
vena cava at angiography arrives in the systemic venous atrium entirely by
way of azygous–inferior vena caval collateral vessels. At angiography in patients with partial superior vena caval obstruction, the systemic venous atrium
fills with radiographic contrast material from both the superior vena cava and
the inferior vena cava.

Using two-dimensional contrast echocardiography, the same flow patterns can be observed in patients with complete, partial, or no superior vena
caval obstruction (Fig. 10-21).[14] Saline is injected into an arm or scalp vein,
while the inferior vena cava, from below the hepatic veins to its junction with
the systemic venous atrium, is imaged from the subcostal long-axis view. Following the saline injection in patients with no superior vena caval obstruction, contrast echoes are seen immediately in the systemic venous atrium
(Fig. 10-22). No contrast echoes are seen in the lower inferior vena cava. However, reflux of contrast echoes into the upper inferior vena cava and hepatic

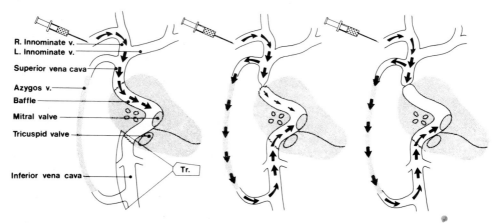

FIG. 10-21. *Diagrammatic representation of three echocardiographic contrast patterns observed in patients following the Mustard operation.* **Left.** *A contrast injection
is made into an arm or scalp vein while the transducer (Tr.) is applied in the subcostal
long-axis plane to image the junction of the inferior vena cava with the systemic venous atrium. In patients with no superior vena caval obstruction, the contrast echoes
(black arrows) fill the systemic venous atrium from above. No contrast echoes are seen
in the lower inferior vena cava.* **Middle.** *In patients with partial superior vena caval
obstruction, contrast echoes are seen filling the systemic venous atrium from above.
Subsequently, contrast echoes are seen in the lower inferior vena cava flowing toward
the systemic venous atrium. These contrast echoes arrived in the inferior vena cava by
way of azygous–inferior vena cava collateral vessels.* **Right.** *In patients with complete
superior vena caval obstruction, the contrast echoes fill the systemic venous atrium
entirely from below by way of azygous–inferior vena cava collateral vessels.*

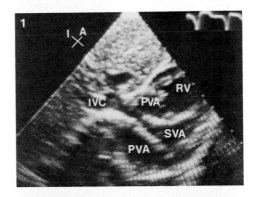

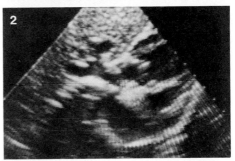

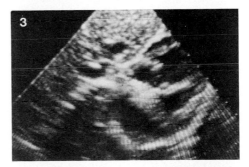

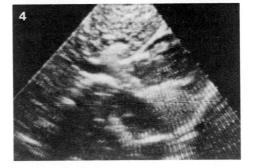

FIG. 10-22. 1. *Contrast echocardiogram in the subcostal long-axis plane from a patient after the Mustard operation. A, anterior; I, inferior; IVC, inferior vena cava; PVA, pulmonary venous atrium; RV, right ventricle; SVA, systemic venous atrium.* **2.** *The contrast echoes fill the systemic venous atrium from above.* **3.** *The contrast echoes are refluxing into the upper inferior vena cava and the hepatic veins. There are no contrast echoes in the inferior vena cava below the hepatic veins.* **4.** *Contrast echoes are seen in the pulmonary venous atrium due to a right-to-left baffle leak.*

veins can be seen during vigorous atrial contraction. Following the saline injection in patients with partial superior vena caval obstruction, contrast echoes are seen first in the systemic venous atrium (Fig. 10-23). During subsequent cardiac cycles, contrast echoes appear in the lower inferior vena cava and flow toward the systemic venous atrium. These contrast echoes reach the lower inferior vena cava by way of azygous–inferior vena cava collateral vessels. Following the contrast injection in patients with complete superior vena caval obstruction, contrast echoes are seen first in the lower inferior vena cava traveling toward the systemic venous atrium (Fig. 4-15). In these patients, there is no opacification of the systemic venous atrium prior to the arrival of contrast echoes in the lower inferior vena cava by way of azygous collaterals.

We have not been successful enough in directly visualizing the area of superior vena caval obstruction to use this approach routinely.

We have examined no patients with inferior vena caval obstruction but believe that inferior vena caval obstruction could be visualized directly in the subcostal planes. We have examined only one patient with pulmonary venous obstruction. On the two-dimensional echocardiogram, the area of pulmonary venous obstruction, which occurred in this patient at the junction of the pulmonary veins with the atrium, could not be imaged directly. However, other findings suggesting pulmonary artery hypertension (dilated, thickened left ventricle) were present.

Chamber Sizes

Following the Mustard operation, the right ventricle remains dilated and hypertrophic in response to its role as the systemic ventricle. The left ventricular posterior wall is usually considerably thinner than the right ventricular anterior wall, and the left ventricular dimensions are much less than the right ventricular dimensions. In the parasternal and subcostal short-axis views, the right ventricle is dominant and circular while the left ventricle is crescent shaped. In the long- and short-axis views, the septum bulges posteriorly into the left ventricle and produces dynamic subpulmonary narrowing. When left ventricular pressures are elevated due to pulmonary vascular obstructive disease, pulmonary venous obstruction, pulmonary stenosis, or a significant residual ventricular septal defect, the left ventricle enlarges and becomes circular and the posterior bulging of the ventricular septum disappears.

Subpulmonary Stenosis

Subpulmonary stenosis occurring after the Mustard operation can be caused by the posterior bulge of the ventricular septum into the left ventricular outflow tract or by the development of an obstructing subpulmonary membrane or a fibromuscular shelf. The parasternal and apical long-axis views are especially useful for detecting subpulmonary stenosis. Frequently, systolic anterior motion of the tip of the anterior mitral valve leaflet can be observed in these views, but this finding cannot be used to differentiate organic from dynamic narrowing.

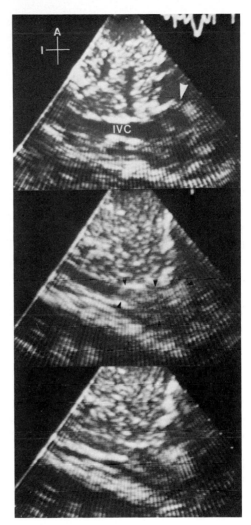

FIG. 10-23. Top. *Subcostal long-axis view prior to contrast injection in a patient after the Mustard procedure with partial superior vena caval obstruction. The white arrow indicates the baffle. A, anterior; I, inferior; IVC, inferior vena cava.* Middle. *Following an arm vein injection, the contrast echoes are seen in the systemic venous atrium and upper inferior vena cava (black arrows). The lower inferior vena cava is free of contrast echoes.* Bottom. *Subsequently, contrast echoes are seen in the lower inferior vena cava traveling toward the systemic venous atrium.*

As significant subpulmonary stenosis develops and the left ventricular pressure becomes elevated, the left ventricle enlarges and the posterior bulge of the ventricular septum disappears. Therefore, the posterior septal bulge is a favorable finding that suggests mild, usually dynamic subpulmonary narrowing.

l-TRANSPOSITION OF THE GREAT ARTERIES

On the two-dimensional echocardiogram, the diagnosis of l-transposition in situs solitus is based on detecting the aorta anterior and to the left of the pulmonary artery and the anatomic right ventricle to the left of the anatomic left

ventricle. The findings that suggest the echocardiographic diagnosis of
l-transposition were discussed in the beginning of this chapter. Further discussion of the diagnosis of l-transposition in situs inversus is included in
Chapter 14.

Because the aortic arch is positioned at the left upper cardiac border in
patients with l-transposition, the suprasternal notch long-axis view can be obtained by positioning the transducer in the left infraclavicular area in a plane
passing between the left nipple and left scapular tip. In this view, the ascending aorta is near the apex of the plane (Fig. 10-24). Usually in l-transposition, the aortic arch cannot be visualized from the suprasternal notch location.

Associated Defects

A high percentage of patients with l-transposition have associated cardiac defects such as pulmonic stenosis, ventricular septal defect, or Ebstein anomaly
of the left-sided atrioventricular valve. In patients with valvar pulmonic stenosis, the pulmonary valve annulus is usually smaller than the aortic valve
annulus in the short-axis views. Poststenotic dilatation of the main pulmonary
artery can be seen in the suprasternal notch views.

In l-transposition, ventricular septal defects can occur in the membranous, muscular, or outlet septum. In some patients with l-transposition, the
ventricular septum can be parallel to the echocardiographic plane and can
cause artifactual echo dropout in the septum. In these cases it can be difficult
to exclude a ventricular septal defect or, in extreme cases, a single ventricle.
Contrast echocardiography and examination of the ventricular septum in multiple planes is essential in differentiating artifactual dropout from a ventricular septal defect.

Ebstein anomaly of the left-sided tricuspid valve is frequently associated
with l-transposition. This defect will be discussed in detail in Chapter 12.

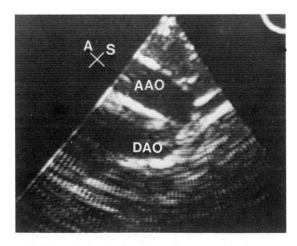

FIG. 10-24. *Long-axis view of the
aortic arch from a patient with
l-transposition. In order to image
the aortic arch, the transducer is
positioned in the left infraclavicular area in a plane passing between the left nipple and left scapular tip. Unlike the standard
long-axis view of the aortic arch in
which the transverse aorta is in
the apex of the plane, the ascending aorta (AAO) in this situation is in the apex of the plane. A,
anterior; DAO, descending aorta;
S, superior.*

Chamber Sizes

In l-transposition with no hemodynamically significant associated defects, the left-sided right ventricle is the dominant ventricle. The right ventricular wall thickness and right ventricular dimensions exceed those of the low pressure left ventricle. The left atrium is larger than the right atrium. In l-transposition with significant pulmonic stenosis, the left ventricle becomes concentrically thickened. In l-transposition with Ebstein anomaly of the left atrioventricular valve, the left atrium is markedly enlarged due to valvar regurgitation and to the presence of the atrialized right ventricle.

REFERENCES

1. Henry WL, Maron BJ, Griffith JM, Redwood DR, Epstein SE: Differential diagnosis of anomalies of the great arteries by real-time two-dimensional echocardiography. Circulation 51: 283, 1975
2. Henry WL, Maron BJ, Griffith JM: Cross-sectional echocardiography in the diagnosis of congenital heart disease: Identification of the relation of the ventricles and great arteries. Circulation 56: 267, 1977
3. Goldberg SJ, Spitaels SEC, de Ville Neuve VH, Ligtrock CM: A controlled evaluation of two-dimensional echo criteria for d-transposition of the great arteries. Circulation 56 (Suppl III): III-41, 1977
4. Maron BJ, Henry WL, Griffith JM, Freedom RM, Kelly DT, Epstein SE: Identification of congenital malformations of the great arteries in infants by real-time two-dimensional echocardiography. Circulation 52: 671, 1975
5. Bierman FZ, Williams RG: Prospective diagnosis of d-transposition of the great arteries in neonates by subxiphoid two-dimensional echocardiography. Circulation 60: 1496, 1979
6. Park SC, Neches WH, Zuberbuhler JR, Mathews RA, Lenox CC, Fricker FJ: Echocardiographic and hemodynamic correlation in transposition of the great arteries. Circulation 57: 291, 1978
7. Nanda NC, Gramiak R, Manning JA, Lipchik EO: Echocardiographic features of subpulmonic obstruction in dextrotransposition of the great vessels. Circulation 51: 515, 1975
8. Aziz KU, Paul MH, Muster AJ: Echocardiographic assessment of the left ventricular outflow tract in d-transposition of the great arteries. Am J Cardiol 41: 543, 1978
9. Bierman FZ, Williams RG: Subxiphoid two-dimensional imaging of the interatrial septum in infants and neonates with congenital heart disease. Circulation 60: 80, 1979
10. Nanda NC, Stewart S, Gramiak R, Manning JA: Echocardiography of the intra-atrial baffle in dextro-transposition of the great vessels. Circulation 51: 1130, 1975
11. Aziz KU, Paul MH, Muster AJ: Echocardiographic localization of interatrial baffle after Mustard's operation for dextro-transposition of the great arteries. Am J Cardiol 38: 67, 1976
12. Silverman NH, Payot M, Stanger P, Rudolph AM: The echocardiographic profile of patients after Mustard's operation. Circulation 58: 1083, 1978

13. Silove ED, Taylor JFN: Hemodynamics after Mustard's operation for transposition of the great arteries. Br Heart J 38: 1037, 1976
14. Silverman NH, Snider AR, Coló J, Ebert PA, Turley K; Superior vena caval obstruction after Mustard's operation: Detection by two-dimensional contrast echocardiography. Circulation 64: 392, 1981

CHAPTER 11

Hypoplastic Left or Right Heart

AORTIC AND MITRAL ATRESIA

The hypoplastic left heart syndrome includes a wide spectrum of anatomic abnormalities. Previous M-mode echocardiographic studies have suggested that the diagnosis of hypoplastic left heart syndrome be made when the left ventricular end-diastolic dimension is less than 9 mm and the aortic root diameter is less than 6 mm.[1,2] With the use of two-dimensional echocardiography,.it is now possible to obtain more detailed anatomic information concerning the size of the left ventricle and ascending aorta and the patency of the aortic and mitral valves in these patients.[3]

In most patients with hypoplastic left heart syndrome, both aortic and mitral valves are atretic or hypoplastic. In these patients, the left ventricle varies in size from slitlike to slightly smaller than normal depending on the degree of hypoplasia of the mitral valve. In patients with mitral atresia and a ventricular septal defect, the ascending aorta and left ventricle can be nearly normal in size if there is a large right-to-left ventricular shunt.

In the parasternal and apical long-axis views, the patency of the aortic and mitral valves can be determined. Usually, an extremely diminutive aorta and a muscle-bound left ventricle with a slitlike cavity are seen (Fig. 11-1). In some patients with a functioning mitral valve, the left ventricular cavity is small but not slitlike (Fig. 11-2). Regardless of its dimensions, the left ventricle is usually stiff and noncontractile. Often, bright echoes are seen arising from areas of fibroelastosis in the endocardium.

The enlarged right atrium, right ventricle, and pulmonary artery can be seen in the parasternal and subcostal short-axis views through the base of the heart (Figs. 11-2 and 11-3). The pulmonary valve is usually densely reflective

189

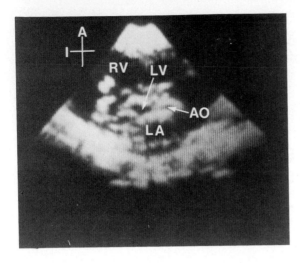

FIG. 11-1. *Parasternal long-axis view from a newborn with aortic and mitral atresia. The ascending aorta (Ao) is diminutive. The left ventricle (LV) has a slitlike cavity and is extremely hypertrophic. The right ventricle (RV) is enlarged. A, anterior; I, inferior; LA, left atrium.*

because of pulmonary artery hypertension. In the short-axis views, the size of the aortic root can be determined, and occasionally, rudimentary aortic valve leaflets can be seen. In some patients, a patent ductus arteriosus can be seen connecting to the descending aorta (Fig. 11-3). In the short-axis views through the left ventricle, the stiff, hypertrophic left ventricle can be imaged (Fig. 11-4).

In the apical and subcostal four-chamber views of patients with aortic and mitral atresia, the left atrium is extremely small and the left ventricle is a rudimentary, slitlike chamber (Fig. 11-5). The right atrium and right ventricle are greatly enlarged. In patients with aortic atresia or hypoplasia and a small, functioning mitral valve, the left ventricular cavity can be larger (Fig. 11-2).

In the suprasternal notch views, the transverse aorta is usually small. The ascending aorta can be threadlike or impossible to image (Fig. 11-6).

Contrast Echocardiography

In many patients with hypoplastic left heart syndrome, there is no right-to-left shunt at the atrial or ventricular level following a peripheral venous contrast injection. In the short-axis view through the base of the heart, contrast echoes frequently can be seen passing from right to left through the patent ductus arteriosus into the descending aorta. Following opacification of the pulmonary artery and patent ductus arteriosus, the ascending aorta fills retrograde with contrast echoes from the descending aorta via the patent ductus arteriosus. In patients with no intracardiac right-to-left shunt, the right-to-left ductal shunt also can be detected by imaging the descending aorta in the subcostal long-axis view during the peripheral venous injection.

Contrast injections made into an umbilical artery catheter positioned in

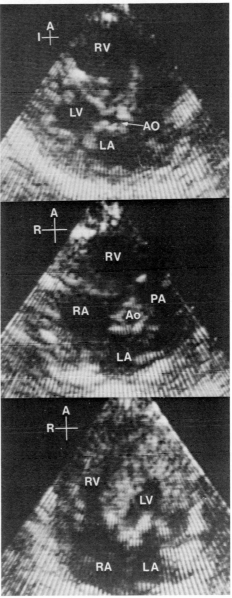

FIG. 11-2. Top. *Parasternal long-axis view from a newborn with aortic atresia and a hypoplastic mitral valve. The ascending aorta (AO) is extremely small. The left ventricle (LV) is hypertrophic but has a larger cavity than the patient in Fig. 11-1. The right ventricle (RV) is enlarged. A, anterior; I, inferior; LA, left atrium.* **Middle.** *Parasternal short-axis view from the same patient. The right atrium (RA), right ventricle (RV), and pulmonary artery (PA) are enlarged, and the small aortic root (Ao) is seen. A, anterior; LA, left atrium; R, right.* **Bottom.** *Apical four-chamber view from the same patient. The left ventricle (LV) is extremely thickened. Bright echoes are seen arising from areas of fibroelastosis in the endocardium. A small, patent mitral valve is present. A, apex; LA, left atrium; R, right; RA, right atrium; RV, right ventricle.*

the descending aorta also demonstrate retrograde filling of the ascending aorta (Fig. 11-7). Following opacification of the ascending aorta in patients with an atretic aortic valve, contrast echoes remain in the ascending aorta for a long time. In patients with a patent aortic valve, contrast echoes are quickly

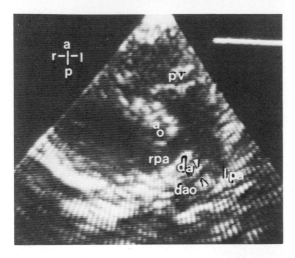

FIG. 11-3. *Parasternal short-axis view from a patient with hypoplastic left heart syndrome. The right heart structures are enlarged and the pulmonary valve (pv) is densely reflective because of pulmonary artery hypertension. A patent ductus arteriosus (da) is seen between the pulmonary artery and descending aorta (dao). a, anterior; ao, aorta; l, left; lpa, left pulmonary artery; p, posterior; r, right; rpa, right pulmonary artery.*

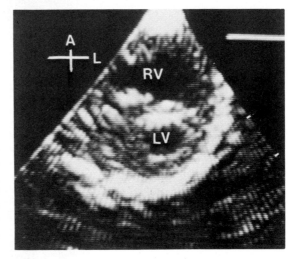

FIG. 11-4. *Parasternal short-axis view through the left ventricle (LV) from the same patient as in Fig. 11-3. The left ventricle is small and hypertrophic. The endocardium is densely reflective. The right ventricle (RV) is enlarged. A, anterior; L, left.*

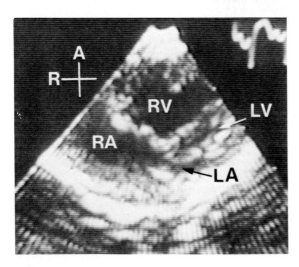

FIG. 11-5. *Apical four-chamber view of a patient with aortic and mitral atresia. A rudimentary, slitlike left ventricle (LV) is seen. The left atrium (LA) is small, and the right atrium (RA) and right ventricle (RV) are enlarged. A, apex; R, right.*

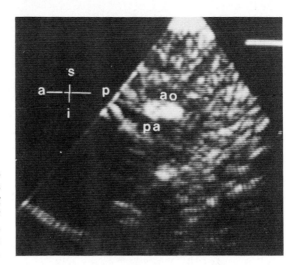

FIG. 11-6. *Suprasternal notch long-axis view from a patient with aortic atresia. The ascending aorta cannot be seen, and the transverse aorta (ao) is small. a, anterior; i, inferior; p, posterior; pa, pulmonary artery; s, superior.*

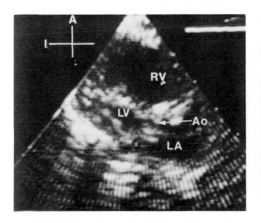 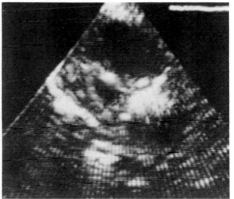

FIG. 11-7. *Contrast injection in the parasternal long-axis view from an infant with aortic atresia.* **Left.** *Prior to the contrast injection, a small left ventricle (LV) and ascending aorta (AO) are seen. A, anterior; I, inferior; LA, left atrium; RV, right ventricle.* **Right.** *Echoes from a contrast injection into an umbilical artery catheter positioned in the descending aorta fill the ascending aorta retrograde. In real time, contrast echoes persisted for a considerable period of time in the ascending aorta because of lack of forward flow from the left ventricle.*

washed out of the ascending aorta by the forward flow from the left ventricle. In the short-axis view, contrast injections made into an umbilical artery catheter in the descending aorta demonstrate filling of the main pulmonary artery from the patent ductus arteriosus followed by retrograde filling of the ascending aorta (see Fig. 4-12).

TRICUSPID ATRESIA

Tricuspid atresia is a rare cause of cyanosis occurring in approximately 1 to 3 percent of patients with congenital heart disease.[4] The characteristic M-mode echocardiographic findings in tricuspid atresia include absence of the tricuspid valve echo, small anterior right ventricular chamber, and a posterior atrioventricular (mitral) valve with large diastolic excursion.[1,5-7] Although the M-mode echocardiogram is extremely useful in the initial evaluation of the critically ill cyanotic newborn, the M-mode echocardiogram does not provide the detailed anatomic information that is necessary prior to palliative or reconstructive surgery. In instances where a structure resembling a tricuspid valve echo has been recorded in a patient with tricuspid atresia, the M-mode echocardiogram has even been misleading.[8,9] Two-dimensional echocardiography provides information on the size and architecture of the right ventricle, the size of the main pulmonary artery and its branches, the ventriculoarterial connections, and the presence of associated cardiac abnormalities.[7,10]

Diagnosis and Classification of Tricuspid Atresia

The diagnosis of tricuspid atresia is made by two-dimensional echocardiography when tricuspid valve leaflets cannot be imaged in any of the standard parasternal, apical, or subcostal planes. The apical four-chamber view, a posterior plane in which both ventricular inlets and the ventricular septum are visualized simultaneously, is most useful for the initial diagnosis of tricuspid atresia (Fig. 11-8). According to Edwards and Burchell, further subclassification of tricuspid atresia into anatomic types depends upon recognizing (1) the ventriculoarterial connections, (2) the presence of pulmonary stenosis or atresia, and (3) the presence of a ventricular septal defect (Table 11-1)[11]

The ventriculoarterial connections (transposed versus normal) can be determined from the parasternal and subcostal short-axis views. In patients with normally related great vessels (type I tricuspid atresia), the pulmonary valve is anterior and to the left of the aortic valve. The right ventricle and pulmonary artery curve anteriorly around the aorta and create a "circle-sausage" appearance in the short-axis views. In patients with transposition (type II), the great vessels have a parallel exit from the heart and are seen in the short-axis views as "double circles."[12] With cranial angulation of the transducer, the bifurcation of the posterior pulmonary artery can be imaged.

The presence of pulmonary atresia or stenosis can be determined from the parasternal and subcostal short-axis views. In patients with no pulmonary stenosis (type IC and IIC), the pulmonary valve annulus and aortic valve annulus are nearly the same size in the short-axis views. In patients with pulmonary stenosis (type IB and IIB), the pulmonary valve annulus is usually considerably smaller than the aortic valve annulus in the short-axis views; also, the main pulmonary artery and its branches are small. In patients with pulmonary atresia (types IA and IIA), an imperforate membrane is usually present in the location normally occupied by the pulmonary valve.

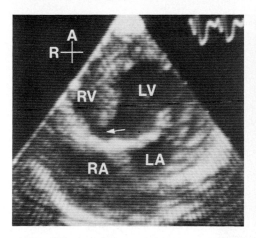 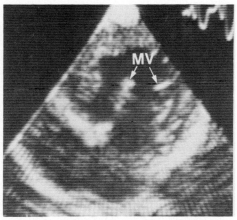

FIG. 11-8. *Apical four-chamber views in systole (**left**) and diastole (**right**) from a patient with type IB tricuspid atresia. Tricuspid valve leaflets are absent, and a dense echo is present in systole and diastole in the area normally occupied by the tricuspid valve. The right ventricle (RV) is extremely small. The right atrium (RA) is enlarged, and the atrial septum is bulging toward the left. A small ventricular septal defect (white arrow) is present. A, apex; LA, left atrium; LV, left ventricle; MV, mitral valve leaflets; R, right.*

TABLE 11-1. ANATOMIC TYPES OF TRICUSPID ATRESIA*

	A	B	C
I (No TGA)	PA Intact ventricular septum	PS Small VSD	No PS Large VSD
II (TGA)	PA Large VSD	PS Large VSD	No PS Large VSD

* Classification by Edwards and Burchell[11]
Abbreviations: PA, pulmonary atresia; PS, pulmonary stenosis; TGA, transposition of the great arteries; VSD, ventricular septal defect

The presence of an intact ventricular septum, small ventricular septal defect, or large ventricular septal defect can be determined from the apical four-chamber view. Patients with a small ventricular septal defect generally have a small right ventricle, and patients with a large ventricular septal defect have a large right ventricle.

Chamber Sizes

In patients with tricuspid atresia, the right ventricular size varies from being either extremely small (Fig. 11-8), small (Fig. 11-9), or slightly smaller than normal (Fig. 11-10). Right ventricular size depends largely upon the amount

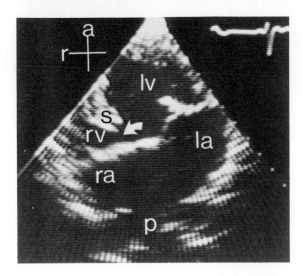

FIG. 11-9. *Apical four-chamber view from a patient with type IIB tricuspid atresia. A large ventricular septal defect is present (white arrow). The right ventricle (rv) is small. a, apex; la, left atrium; lv, left ventricle; p, pulmonary veins; r, right; ra, right atrium; s, septum.*

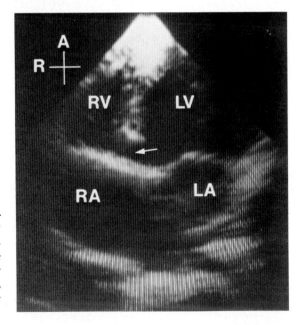

FIG. 11-10. *Apical four-chamber view from a patient with type IC tricuspid atresia. A large ventricular septal defect is present (white arrow). The right ventricle (RV) is slightly smaller than normal. A, apex; LA, left atrium; LV, left ventricle; R, right; RA, right atrium.*

of right-to-left shunting at the ventricular level. Overall right ventricular size can be estimated from two views—the apical four-chamber view to assess the trabeculated portion of the right ventricle and the parasternal short-axis view to assess the right ventricular outflow area.

The left ventricle is usually a large, dilated chamber that can be seen in several echocardiographic planes. In the short-axis and four-chamber views, the right atrium is also enlarged and the atrial septum bulges toward the left (Fig. 11-8). Pulmonary artery size is variable and can be assessed from the short-axis and suprasternal notch views.

Associated Defects

The two-dimensional echocardiogram is extremely useful in the detection of associated cardiac defects. Mitral valve prolapse is present in approximately 66 percent of patients with tricuspid atresia.[6] Enlargement of the coronary sinus in patients with tricuspid atresia is a frequent finding that can be caused by right atrial hypertension or anomalous venous return to the coronary sinus. Bharati and colleagues reported finding at autopsy a left superior vena cava to coronary sinus in 13.4 percent of type I tricuspid atresia patients.[13]

Contrast Echocardiography

Following a peripheral venous contrast injection, patients with tricuspid atresia have a large right-to-left atrial shunt. In the four-chamber views in patients with a ventricular septal defect, contrast echoes often can be seen in the right ventricle following opacification of the left ventricle.

PULMONARY ATRESIA

The two basic types of pulmonary atresia are (1) pulmonary atresia with an intact ventricular septum and (2) pulmonary atresia with a conotruncal defect. The latter type of pulmonary atresia was discussed in Chapter 9. In most cases of pulmonary atresia with an intact septum, the obstruction is due to an imperforate pulmonary valve.[14] In the parasternal and subcostal short-axis views, the imperforate valve appears as a thick band of echoes (Fig. 11-11). The

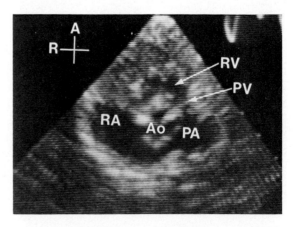

FIG. 11-11. *Parasternal short-axis view through the base of the heart from a patient with pulmonary atresia and an intact ventricular septum. The pulmonary valve (PV) is unperforated. The right ventricle (RV) is hypertrophic and small. The right atrium (RA) is enlarged. The main pulmonary artery (PA) is of fair size. A, anterior; Ao, aorta; R, right.*

M-mode echocardiogram taken from the area of the imperforate membrane shows an echo with a sine-wave motion but no evidence of a semilunar valve opening or closure. In the short-axis views in patients with isolated pulmonary atresia, the right ventricular infundibulum can be normal or obstructed and the pulmonary arteries can vary in size from normal to hypoplastic (Fig. 11-11). Branch pulmonary artery size can also be determined from the suprasternal notch views.

Isolated pulmonary atresia has been classified into two types based on the size of the right ventricle.[15] In type I the right ventricular cavity is diminutive, and the tricuspid valve is competent. In type II, the right ventricular cavity is normal sized, and there are moderate-to-massive amounts of tricuspid insufficiency. The right ventricular thickness and cavity dimensions can be assessed from the long-axis, short-axis, and four-chamber views. In type I pulmonary atresia the right ventricular cavity is often slitlike on the echocardiogram, and the tricuspid valve is small and extremely thickened (Figs. 11-11 to 11-13). In type II pulmonary atresia the right ventricle is normal sized, and the tricuspid valve leaflets often have an Ebstein-type deformity.[16] The septal leaflet arises normally from the tricuspid annulus, but a fairly large part of the basal portion of the leaflet remains unseparated from the ventricular septum.[14] On the apical four-chamber view, this creates the appearance of leaflet insertion low in the ventricle (see Chapter 12). In both types of pulmonary atresia, the right atrium is enlarged and the atrial septum bulges prominently towards the left (Fig. 11-13).

Contrast Echocardiography

With contrast injections into an umbilical artery catheter positioned in the descending aorta, it is often possible to demonstrate retrograde filling of the pul-

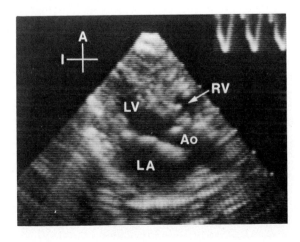

FIG. 11-12. *Parasternal long-axis view from the same patient as in Fig. 11-11. A hypertrophic right ventricle (RV) with a small cavity can be seen. The ventricular septum is intact. A, anterior; Ao, aorta; I, inferior; LA, left atrium; LV, left ventricle.*

monary artery from the patent ductus arteriosus. With peripheral venous contrast echocardiography, most patients with pulmonary atresia have a large right-to-left atrial shunt. In addition, contrast echoes can often be seen filling the lower inferior vena cava and hepatic veins during systole because of tricuspid insufficiency. With a peripheral venous injection, contrast echoes do not flow forward from the right ventricle into the pulmonary artery. Opacification of the pulmonary artery occurs later in a retrograde fashion by way of bronchial collaterals or a patent ductus arteriosus (see Fig. 9-9).

Echocardiography in the Postoperative Patient

Following pulmonary valvotomy or patch reconstruction of the right ventricular outflow tract, the two-dimensional echocardiogram is useful for serial assessment of the right ventricular and pulmonary artery size. The right ventricle can be evaluated from several views. The suprasternal notch views are especially useful in assessing pulmonary artery size. Patients who have undergone pulmonary valvotomy or placement of an outflow tract patch frequently have signs of pulmonary insufficiency on the two-dimensional echocardiogram. These signs include dilated right ventricle, paradoxical septal motion, vigorous right ventricular ejection, and vigorous pulmonary artery pulsations. Following reconstructive surgery, the persistence of a right-to-left atrial shunt during contrast echocardiography usually indicates either (1) residual significant right ventricular outflow obstruction, (2) a noncompliant right ventricle, or (3) significant tricuspid stenosis.

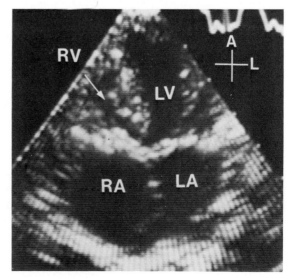

FIG. 11-13. *Apical four-chamber view from the same patient as in Figs. 11-11 and 11-12. A hypertrophic right ventricle (RV) with a small cavity is seen. The ventricular septum is intact. The right atrium (RA) is enlarged, and the atrial septum is bulging towards the left. In real time, a small, thickened tricuspid valve could be seen. A, apex; L, left; LA, left atrium; LV, left ventricle.*

REFERENCES

1. Meyer RA, Kaplan S: Echocardiography in the diagnosis of hypoplasia of the left or right ventricles in the neonate. Circulation 46: 55, 1972

2. Farooki ZQ Henry JG, Green EW: Echocardiographic spectrum of the hypoplastic left heart syndrome: A clinicopathologic correlation in 19 newborns. Am J Cardiol 38: 337, 1976

3. Lange LW, Sahn DJ, Allen HD, Ovitt TW, Goldberg SJ: The utility of cross-sectional echocardiography in the evaluation of hypoplastic left ventricle syndrome—echocardiographic/angiographic/anatomic correlations. Pediatr Cardiol 1: 287, 1980

4. Nadas AS, Fyler DC: Pediatric Cardiology. Philadelphia, Saunders, 1972, pp. 679–683

5. Chesler E, Joffe HS, Vecht R, Beck W, Schrire V: Ultrasound cardiography in single ventricle and the hypoplastic left and right heart syndromes. Circulation 42: 123, 1970

6. Seward JB, Tajik AJ, Hagler DJ, Ritter DG: Echocardiographic spectrum of tricuspid atresia. Mayo Clin Proc 53: 100, 1978

7. Pouget B, Tynan M, Roudaut R, Choussat A, Dallocchio M, Fontan F: Echocardiographic studies in patients with tricuspid atresia or single ventricle before and after Fontan procedure. In Echocardiology, CT Lancée, ed. Boston, Martinus Nijhoff, 1979, p. 335

8. Silverman NH, Payot M, Stanger P: Simulated tricuspid valve echoes in tricuspid atresia. Am Heart J 95: 761, 1978

9. Takahashi O, Eshaghpour E, Kotler MN: Tricuspid and pulmonic valve echoes in tricuspid and pulmonary atresia. Chest 76: 437, 1979

10. Beppu S, Nimura Y, Tamai M, Nagata S, Matsuo H, Kawashima Y, Kozuka T, Sakakibara H: Two-dimensional echocardiography in diagnosing tricuspid atresia: Differentiation from other hypoplastic right heart syndromes and common atrioventricular canal. Br Heart J 40: 1174, 1978

11. Edwards JE, Burchell HB: Congenital tricuspid atresia: A classification. Med Clin North Am 33: 1177, 1949

12. Henry WL, Maron BJ, Griffith JM, Redwood DR, Epstein SE: Differential diagnosis of anomalies of the great arteries by real-time two-dimensional echocardiography. Circulation 51: 283, 1975

13. Bharati S, McAllister HA Jr, Tatooles CJ, Miller RA, Weinberg M Jr, Bucheleres HG, Lev M: Anatomic variations in underdeveloped right ventricle related to tricuspid atresia and stenosis. J Thorac Cardiovasc Surg 72: 383, 1976

14. Goor DA, Lillehei CW: Congenital Malformations of the Heart. New York, Grune and Stratton, 1975, pp. 325–328

15. Greenwold WE, Dushane JW, Burchell HB, Bruner A, Edwards JE: Congenital pulmonary atresia with intact ventricular septum: Two anatomic types. Proc 29th Scientific Session, Am Heart Association, October, 1956, p. 51

16. Lewis BS, Amitai N, Simcha A, Merin G, Gotsman MS: Echocardiographic diagnosis of pulmonary atresia with intact ventricular septum. Am Heart J 97: 92, 1979

CHAPTER 12

Other Cyanotic Lesions

EBSTEIN ANOMALY OF THE TRICUSPID VALVE

Ebstein anomaly consists of a downward displacement of the septal and posterior leaflets of the tricuspid valve away from the annulus fibrosus. This displacement results in atrialization of the proximal portion of the right ventricle, a reduction in size of the functioning right ventricle, and tricuspid insufficiency. The anterior tricuspid valve leaflet is usually thickened and redundant and can cause right ventricular outflow obstruction. Variations in the degree of downward displacement of the tricuspid valve lead to a wide spectrum of anatomic abnormalities in patients with Ebstein anomaly.

Two-dimensional echocardiography provides a method for the accurate diagnosis of Ebstein anomaly.[1-3] The most useful view for the initial diagnosis of Ebstein anomaly is the apical four-chamber view (Fig. 12-1). In this view the septal leaflet of the tricuspid valve usually is displaced toward the ventricular apex, and the anterior leaflet of the tricuspid valve arises normally from the annulus fibrosus. The tricuspid valve leaflets are thickened and deformed, and the anterior tricuspid valve leaflet is redundant. The portion of the right ventricle between the atrioventricular groove and the displaced tricuspid valve is the atrialized right ventricle. The true functioning right ventricle is that portion of the right ventricle that is located inferior to the displaced tricuspid valve. On the apical four-chamber view, there frequently is evidence of right ventricular volume overload and paradoxical septal motion. In some patients, because of the dilatation of the right atrium and right ventricle and the resultant posterior and lateral displacement of the left ventricle, it may be difficult to obtain adequate apical views.

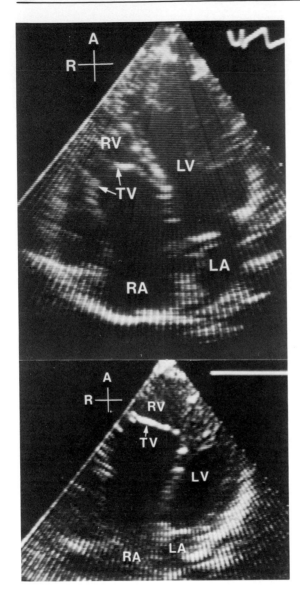

FIG. 12-1. Top. *Apical four-chamber view from a patient with Ebstein anomaly of the tricuspid valve (TV). The septal leaflet of the tricuspid valve is displaced downward toward the cardiac apex. The anterior (right lateral) leaflet attaches normally to the annulus fibrosus. The moderator band can be seen in the apex of the right ventricle (RV). The atrialized right ventricle is located between the atrioventricular groove and the displaced tricuspid valve. The functioning right ventricle is located inferior to the displaced tricuspid valve. A, apex; LA, left atrium; LV, left ventricle; R, right; RA, right atrium.* **Bottom.** *Apical four-chamber view from a different patient with Ebstein anomaly of the tricuspid valve (TV). Abbreviations are the same as above.*

In the apical four-chamber view in the normal heart, the distances from the mitral valve to the cardiac apex and from the tricuspid valve to the cardiac apex are nearly equal. The ratio between the mitral valve–apex distance and the tricuspid valve–apex distance averages 1.1 in normal patients. In patients with Ebstein anomaly, the ratio between the mitral–apex distance and the tricuspid–apex distance is always greater than 1.5.[3]

In the parasternal and apical long-axis views, the dilated right ventricle and the thickened, redundant anterior tricuspid valve leaflet can be seen rotated toward the patient's left (Fig. 12-2). The abnormal attachments of the

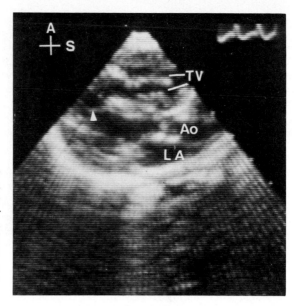

FIG. 12-2. *Parasternal long-axis view from a patient with Ebstein anomaly of the tricuspid valve (TV). A large redundant anterior leaflet can be seen. The right ventricle is dilated. An additional muscular ventricular septal defect (arrow) can be seen. A, anterior; Ao, aorta; LA, left atrium; S, superior.*

septal and posterior leaflets are seldom seen in this view. The echocardiographic findings in the long-axis views do not distinguish Ebstein anomaly from other conditions causing chronic right ventricular volume overload.

In the parasternal and subcostal short-axis views, the displacement of the septal leaflet of the tricuspid valve into the right ventricular outflow tract can be seen (Fig. 12-3);[2] however, the exact attachments of the tricuspid valve leaflets may be difficult to image. Evidence of right ventricular volume overload and right atrial enlargement is usually present in the short-axis views.

In patients with l-transposition with ventricular inversion, Ebstein anomaly of the left-sided tricuspid valve frequently occurs. In the apical four-chamber view in these patients, the anatomic right ventricle can be seen to the left of the anatomic left ventricle (Fig. 12-4). The left-sided tricuspid valve can be seen positioned closer to the cardiac apex than normal (see Chapter 10).

Contrast Echocardiography

Patients with Ebstein anomaly frequently have a right-to-left atrial shunt even when the oxygen saturation is normal. Contrast echocardiography in the apical and subcostal four-chamber views can be used to detect right-to-left atrial shunting through an open foramen ovale or an associated atrial septal defect. In addition, tricuspid insufficiency can be detected during contrast echocardiography by imaging the inferior vena cava in the subcostal long-axis view. In patients with tricuspid insufficiency, contrast echoes are seen in the inferior vena cava and hepatic veins during systole.[4] It is important to note that contrast echoes are normally seen in the inferior vena cava and hepatic veins during diastole due to vigorous atrial contraction.

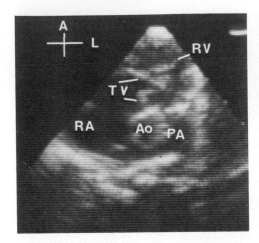
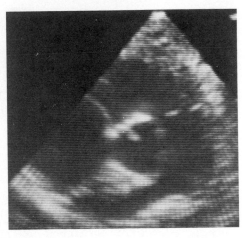

FIG. 12-3. **Left.** *Parasternal short-axis view from a patient with Ebstein anomaly. (A normal short-axis view is shown for camparison,* **right.**) *The septal leaflet of the tricuspid valve (TV) is displaced toward the right ventricular outflow tract. The anterior tricuspid valve leaflet is large and redundant. The right atrium (RA) is dilated. A, anterior; Ao, aorta; L, left; PA, pulmonary artery; RV, right ventricle.*

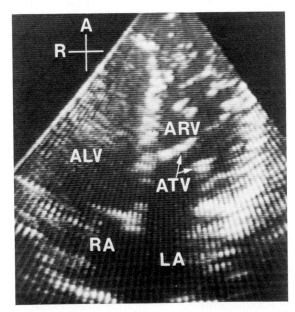

FIG. 12-4. *Ebstein anomaly of the left-sided anatomic tricuspid valve (ATV) in a patient with l-transposition and ventricular inversion. The tricuspid valve is positioned closer to the cardiac apex than usual. A, apex; ALV, anatomic left ventricle; ARV, anatomic right ventricle; LA, left atrium; R, right; RA, right atrium.*

Associated Defects

Associated atrial and ventricular septal defects are commonly seen in patients with Ebstein anomaly on the two-dimensional echocardiographic examination (Fig. 12-5). Also, tricuspid valve prolapse can be detected in the apical four-chamber view and the parasternal short-axis view. The presence of pul-

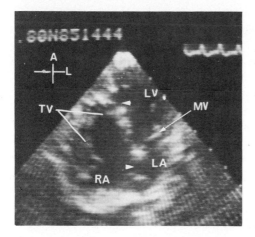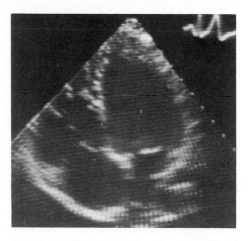

FIG. 12-5. Left. *Apical four-chamber view from a patient with Ebstein anomaly of the tricuspid valve (TV). (A normal apical four-chamber view is shown for comparison,* **right**.*) The tricuspid valve septal leaflet is displaced downward toward the cardiac apex. The anterior leaflet is large and redundant and arises normally from the annulus fibrosus. Additional atrial and ventricular septal defects (arrows) are seen. A, apex; L, left; LA, left atrium; LV, left ventricle; MV, mitral valve; RA, right atrium.*

monary stenosis and the size of the main pulmonary artery and its branches can be detected best in the short-axis views.

TOTAL ANOMALOUS PULMONARY VENOUS RETURN

In patients with total anomalous pulmonary venous return, the pulmonary veins usually converge to form a common pulmonary venous chamber posterior to the left atrium. The common pulmonary venous chamber drains most often to the coronary sinus or to the superior vena cava by way of a left vertical vein and innominate vein. Less often, the common pulmonary venous chamber drains directly to the right atrium or to the hepatic–portal system. M-mode echocardiographic features of total anomalous pulmonary venous return include evidence of right ventricular volume overload and identification of an echo-free space (the common pulmonary venous chamber) behind the left atrium.[5-7]

On the two-dimensional echocardiogram, the exact location of drainage of the common pulmonary venous chamber can be better appreciated.[8] In patients with total anomalous pulmonary venous return, the right atrium, right ventricle, and pulmonary arteries are enlarged on the two-dimensional echocardiogram; also, the right ventricular anterior wall is thickened, and the pulmonary valve is densely reflective suggesting pulmonary artery hypertension. There is usually no appreciable movement of the ventricular septum. The left atrium and left ventricle can be normal or diminished in size.

Frequently, the common pulmonary venous chamber can be seen posterior and superior to the left atrium (Figs. 12-6 and 12-7). In order to visualize the thin wall separating the common pulmonary venous chamber from the left atrium, careful attention must be given to gain and reject settings. Failure to visualize a separate common pulmonary venous chamber does not exclude the diagnosis of total anomalous pulmonary venous return.

In total anomalous pulmonary venous return to the coronary sinus, it is often possible to image directly the connection of the common pulmonary venous chamber to the coronary sinus and right atrium. The confluence of the pulmonary veins with the coronary sinus and right atrium can be seen in the parasternal short-axis view and in the. apical four-chamber view (Fig. 12-7). Evidence of an enlarged coronary sinus can also be seen in other echocardiographic planes.

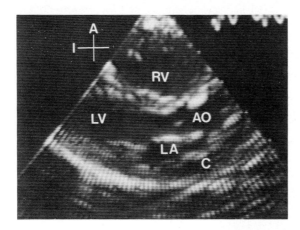

FIG. 12-6. *Parasternal long-axis view from an infant with total anomalous pulmonary venous return to the coronary sinus. The common pulmonary venous chamber (C) is seen posterior and superior to the left atrium (LA) and separated from it by a thin wall. The right ventricle (RV) is enlarged. A, anterior; AO, aorta; I, inferior; LV, left ventricle.*

FIG. 12-7. *Apical four-chamber view from the same patient as in Fig. 12-6. The pulmonary venous confluence (pv) is connected to the right atrium (ra) by a dilated coronary sinus. It is not possible to determine with certainty where the pulmonary venous confluence ends and the coronary sinus begins. The right atrium and right ventricle (rv) are enlarged, and the right ventricle is apex forming. a, apex; la, left atrium; lv, left ventricle; r, right.*

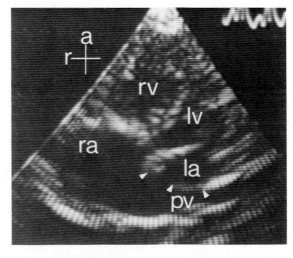

In total anomalous pulmonary venous return to the superior vena cava by way of the left vertical vein and innominate vein, a dilated innominate vein can be seen in cross section in the suprasternal notch long-axis view (Fig. 12-8). In the suprasternal notch short-axis view, the entire connection from the common pulmonary venous chamber to the superior vena cava can be seen as a large vascular collar surrounding the transverse aorta (Fig. 12-9).

In patients with total anomalous pulmonary venous return to the hepatic–portal system, the common pulmonary vein can often be followed in the subcostal views to its site of drainage below the diaphragm. We have had less

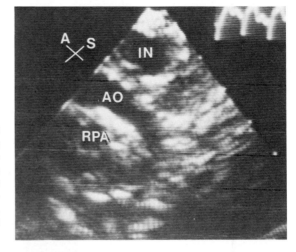

FIG. 12-8. *Suprasternal notch long-axis view from an infant with total anomalous pulmonary venous return to the superior vena cava by way of a left vertical vein and innominate vein. The innominate vein (IN) is markedly dilated. A, anterior; AO, aorta; RPA, right pulmonary artery; S, superior.*

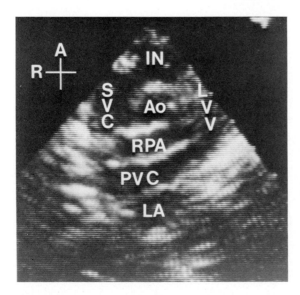

FIG. 12-9. *Suprasternal notch short-axis view from an infant with supradiaphragmatic total anomalous pulmonary venous return. The pulmonary venous confluence (PVC) is superior to the small left atrium (LA) and connects to a left vertical vein (LVV), which drains via the innominate vein (IN) to the superior vena cava (SVC). A, anterior; Ao, aorta; R, right; RPA, right pulmonary artery.*

success in visualizing the exact site of drainage in patients with total anomalous pulmonary venous return directly to the right atrium or superior vena cava.

Patients with total anomalous pulmonary venous return have an obligatory right-to-left atrial shunt that can be seen during peripheral venous contrast echocardiography. Following the contrast injection, all four cardiac chambers and both great vessels are opacified by contrast echoes because of the obligatory right-to-left atrial shunt and forward flow in the left heart. Since contrast echoes are filtered completely in the pulmonary capillary bed, the only structure remaining free of contrast echoes is the common pulmonary venous chamber. This factor can be helpful in verifying the location of the common pulmonary venous chamber.

SINGLE VENTRICLE

The term single ventricle describes a variety of complex congenital malformations characterized by absence of the posterior or inlet portion of the ventricular septum.[9] There have been several reports of the M-mode echocardiographic findings in patients with single ventricle[10-13]; however, the variations in great vessel origin and in atrioventricular valve morphology and attachments are best imaged by two-dimensional echocardiography.

In the normal heart, the inlet septum separates the atrioventricular valves and runs to the crux cordis on the posterior surface of the heart.[9] The apical four-chamber view, a posterior plane which passes through both atrioventricular valves and the posterior inlet septum, is most useful for making the initial diagnosis of single ventricle. In this view in patients with single ventricle, the inlet septum is absent (Fig. 12-10). Occasionally, absence of the inlet

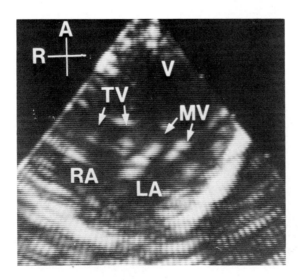

FIG. 12-10. *Apical four-chamber view from a patient with single ventricle (V). The tricuspid and mitral valves (TV and MV) are seen with no intervening ventricular septum. A, apex; LA, left atrium; R, right; RA, right atrium.*

septum can be seen in other views such as the subcostal four-chamber view and the apical long-axis view (Fig. 12-11). More often, remnants of the trabecular and infundibular septa can be seen in the other echocardiographic planes (Fig. 12-12). These structures are anterior septa that do not run to the posterior crux cordis and, therefore, should not be mistaken for the inlet septum. In the apical four-chamber view in some patients, a large papillary muscle arises from the apex of the ventricle and can mimic the appearance of a ventricular septum. Careful examination of the heart in several echocardiographic planes usually resolves this problem.

Single ventricle can occur with two atrioventricular valves, a common atrioventricular valve, a straddling atrioventricular valve, or absence of one atrioventricular valve.[9] Most commonly, two atrioventricular valves empty into the single ventricle. In several echocardiographic planes (especially the short-axis and four-chamber views), the two atrioventricular valves with no intervening septum can be seen communicating with the single ventricle (Fig. 12-10). In the apical four-chamber view in some patients, absence of the right or left atrioventricular valve can be seen (Fig. 12-13). The four-chamber view is also useful for visualizing a common atrioventricular valve.

Single ventricle can occur with or without a rudimentary chamber. The rudimentary chamber can be anterior, left sided, or right sided. If one or both arteries arise primarily from the rudimentary chamber, it is termed an outflow chamber. If neither great artery arises from the rudimentary chamber (both great arteries arise from the main ventricle), it is termed a trabeculated pouch.[9] In the most common type of single ventricle, there is an anterior outlet chamber that gives rise to an anterior transposed aorta. Anterior outlet chambers are best visualized in the parasternal long- and short-axis views (Figs. 12-12 and 12-14). Anterior outlet chambers cannot be visualized in the apical four-chamber view because it is a posterior plane; occasionally, however, right-sided or left-sided rudimentary chambers can be seen in the apical four-chamber view (Fig. 12-13).

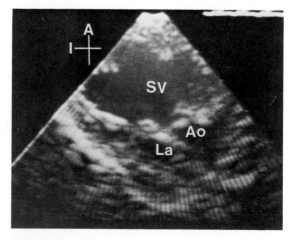

FIG. 12-11. *Apical long-axis view from a patient with single ventricle (SV) and normally related great vessels. There is no evidence of a ventricular septum. The posterior aorta (Ao) arises from the main chamber. The outlet chamber cannot be seen in this view. A, anterior; I, inferior; La, left atrium.*

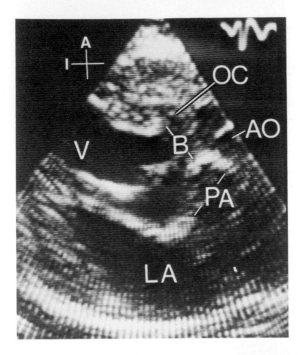

FIG. 12-12. *Parasternal long-axis view from a patient with single ventricle (V), an anterior outlet chamber (OC), and transposition of the great arteries. The anterior aorta (AO) arises from the outlet chamber. The posterior pulmonary artery (PA) arises from the main chamber. The outlet chamber communicates with the main ventricle by way of a bulboventricular foramen (B). A, anterior; I, inferior; LA, left atrium.*

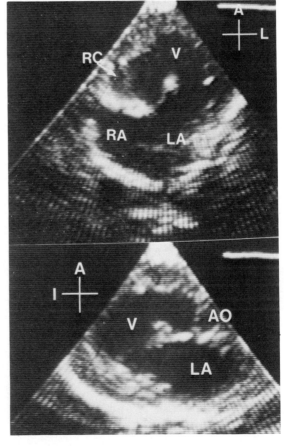

FIG. 12-13. **Top.** *Apical four-chamber view from a patient with single ventricle (V) and absence of the right atrioventricular valve. A right-sided rudimentary chamber (RC) can be seen in this view. A, apex; L, left; LA, left atrium; RA, right atrium.* **Bottom.** *Parasternal long-axis view from the same patient. The aorta (AO) arises from the main ventricle (V). The rudimentary chamber is right-sided rather than anterior and, therefore, could not be seen in this view. A, anterior; I, inferior; LA, left atrium.*

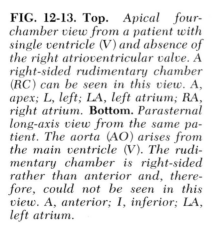

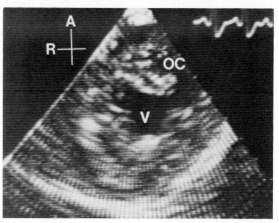

FIG. 12-14. *Parasternal short-axis view from the same patient as in Fig. 12-12. The main ventricle (V) is seen in cross section. The outlet chamber (OC) is anterior and slightly leftward, and the bulboventricular foramen is seen between the ventricle and outlet chamber. A, anterior; R, right.*

In patients with single ventricle, the ventriculoarterial connections can be concordant (aorta from main chamber, pulmonary artery from outlet chamber), discordant or transposed (pulmonary artery from main chamber, aorta from outlet chamber), double outlet from the main chamber or the outlet chamber, or single outlet (truncus arteriosus, pulmonary atresia, aortic atresia).[9] The parasternal and subcostal short-axis views (Fig. 12-15) are most helpful for determining whether the great arteries are normally related, transposed, or in double outlet position (see Chapters 9 and 10). The parasternal

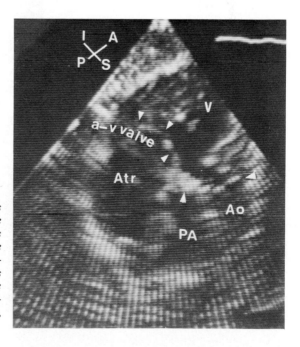

FIG. 12-15. *Subcostal short-axis view from a patient with single ventricle (V). Both great vessels arise from the main ventricle. The aorta (Ao) is anterior to the pulmonary artery (PA). The arrows indicate the atrioventricular valve and the semilunar valves. A, anterior; Atr, atrium; I, inferior; P, posterior; S, superior.*

long-axis view (Fig. 12-12) and the short-axis sweep from the base to the apex of the heart are helpful in determining whether a great artery arises from the outlet chamber or the main chamber.

STRADDLING TRICUSPID VALVE

In patients with straddling tricuspid valve, the tricuspid valve overrides a large ventricular septal defect and opens into both ventricles. Chordae tendinae of the tricuspid valve attach into both ventricles. The right ventricle may be normal in size or underdeveloped, and the atrial and ventricular septa are malaligned.[14]

The apical four-chamber view, which visualizes both atrioventricular valves and the cardiac septa simultaneously, is most useful for the initial diagnosis of tricuspid valve straddle (Figs. 12-16 and 12-17). In this view, the

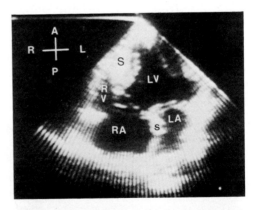

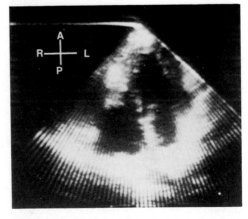

FIG. 12-16 *Apical four-chamber views in systole (**top**) and diastole (**bottom**) from a patient with a straddling tricuspid valve. There is malalignment of the atrial and ventricular septa (S). The right ventricle (RV) is underdeveloped. A, anterior; L, left; LA, left atrium; LV, left ventricle; P, posterior; R, right; RA, right atrium.*

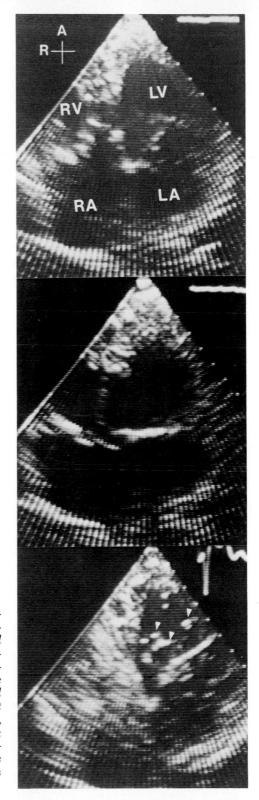

FIG. 12-17. *Four-chamber views in diastole (**top**) and systole (**middle**) from a patient with straddling tricuspid valve and a ventricular septal defect. The ventricular septum and atrial septum are malaligned. The tricuspid valve overrides the ventricular septum and has chordal attachments to both ventricles. The right ventricle (RV) is underdeveloped. A, apex; LA, left atrium; LV, left ventricle; R, right; RA, right atrium. **Bottom.** A peripheral venous contrast injection shows contrast echoes (arrows) passing from the right atrium to the left ventricle.*

malalignment of the atrial and ventricular septa and the malalignment of the tricuspid valve and the ventricular septum can be seen; however, attachments of the tricuspid valve to the left ventricle should be imaged before the diagnosis of tricuspid valve straddle is made. Contrast echocardiography in the apical four-chamber view can be used to show the right-to-left shunt from the right atrium to the left ventricle (Fig. 12-17).

REFERENCES

1. Matsumoto M, Matsuo H, Nagata S, Hamanaka Y, Fujita T, Kawashima V, Nimura Y, Abe H: Visualization of Ebstein's anomaly of the tricuspid valve by two-dimensional and standard echocardiography. Circulation 53: 69, 1976
2. Hirschklau MJ, Sahn DJ, Hagan AD, Williams DE, Friedman WF: Cross-sectional echocardiographic features of Ebstein's anomaly of the tricuspid valve. Am J Cardiol 40: 400, 1977
3. Ports TA, Silverman NH, Schiller NB: Two-dimensional echocardiographic assessment of Ebstein's anomaly. Circulation 58: 336, 1978
4. Lieppe W, Behar V, Scallion R, Kisslo J: Detection of tricuspid regurgitation with two-dimensional echocardiography and peripheral vein injections. Circulation 57: 128, 1978
5. Paquet M, Gutgesell H: Echocardiographic features of total anomalous pulmonary venous connection. Circulation: 51: 599, 1975
6. Orsmond GS, Ruttenberg HD, Bessinger FB, Moller JH: Echocardiographic features of total anomalous pulmonary venous connection to the coronary sinus. Am J Cardiol 41: 597, 1978
7. Aziz KU, Paul MH, Bharati S, Lev M, Shannon K: Echocardiographic features of total anomalous pulmonary venous drainage into the coronary sinus. Am J Cardiol 42: 108, 1978
8. Sahn DJ, Allen HD, Lange LW, Goldberg SJ: Cross-sectional echocardiographic diagnosis of the sites of total anomalous pulmonary venous drainage. Circulation 60: 1317, 1979
9. Anderson RH, Wilkinson JL, Macartney FJ, Tynan MJ, Shinebourne EA, Quero-Jimenez M, Becker AE: Classification and terminology of primitive ventricle. In Paediatric Cardiology 1977, RH Anderson, EA Shinebourne, eds. Edinburgh, Churchill-Livingstone, 1978, pp. 311-322
10. Felner JM, Brewer DB, Franch RH: Echocardiographic manifestations of single ventricle. Am J Cardiol 38: 80, 1976
11. Seward JB, Tajik AJ, Hagler DJ, Ritter DG: Contrast echocardiography in single or common ventricle. Circulation 55: 513, 1977
12. Beardshaw JA, Gibson DG, Pearson MC, Upton MT, Anderson RH: Echocardiographic diagnosis of primitive ventricle with two atrioventricular valves. Br Heart J 39: 266, 1977
13. Bini RM, Bloom KR, Culham JAG, Freedom RM, Williams CM, Rowe RD: The reliability and practicality of single crystal echocardiography in the evaluation of single ventricle. Circulation 57: 269, 1978
14. Milo S, Ho SY, Macartney FJ, Wilkinson JL, Becker AE, Wenink ACG, Gittenberger De Groot AC, Anderson RH: Straddling and overriding atrioventricular valves: Morphology and classification. Am J Cardiol 44: 1122, 1979

CHAPTER 13

Postoperative Patients

PERICARDIAL AND PLEURAL EFFUSIONS

In pediatric patients, pericardial effusions commonly occur following cardiac surgery and also in patients with infections, congestive heart failure, renal disease, hypothyroidism, and juvenile rheumatoid arthritis. On the echocardiogram, pericardial effusions appear as an echo-free space between the epicardium and the pericardium.[1] Effusions can occur anteriorly, posteriorly, or both. Although most effusions can be detected by M-mode echocardiography, two-dimensional echocardiography provides additional information concerning the total spatial distribution of the fluid and the presence of fluid loculations.

On the two-dimensional echocardiogram, pericardial effusions should be examined from every echocardiographic view in order to determine the total area of the fluid (Figs. 13-1 to 13-3). Posterior pericardial effusions occur between the epicardium and the posterior pericardium. The posterior pericardial echo is identified as the brightest echo in the far field and the last echo to disappear as the gains are decreased. Anterior pericardial effusions occur between the epicardium and the anterior pericardium; however, the anterior pericardium may be impossible to visualize as a separate structure from the anterior chest wall. In patients with chronic pericardial effusions, strands or fibrinous material often can be seen within the pericardial fluid (Figs. 13-4 and 13-5).

The exact volume of pericardial fluid usually cannot be determined from the echocardiogram.[2] In general, effusions that occur both anteriorly and posteriorly are large effusions. Also, patients in whom the heart has a dramatic "swinging" motion within the fluid-filled pericardium have large effusions.[3]

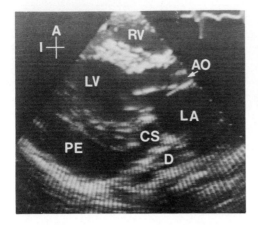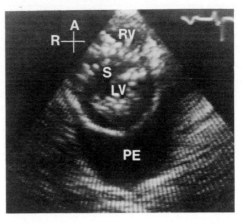

FIG. 13-1. Left. *Parasternal long-axis view from a patient with a moderate-sized pericardial effusion (PE) following closure of a ventricular septal defect. The large echo-free space between the epicardium and posterior pericardium represents the effusion. There is no pericardial fluid anteriorly. A, anterior; AO, aorta; CS, coronary sinus; D, descending aorta; I, inferior; LA, left atrium; LV, left ventricle; RV, right ventricle.* **Right.** *Parasternal short-axis view from the same patient showing the sizable posterior pericardial effusion (PE). A, anterior; LV, left ventricle; R, right; RV, right ventricle; S, septum.*

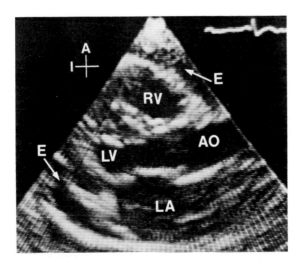

FIG. 13-2. *Parasternal long-axis view from a patient with a large pericardial effusion (E) following cardiac surgery. The effusion extends anteriorly and posteriorly. A, anterior; AO, aorta; I, inferior; LA, left atrium; LV, left ventricle; RV, right ventricle.*

Right ventricular compression (a markedly diminished right ventricular end-diastolic dimension at expiration) has been reported in patients with cardiac tamponade.[4] However, in patients with a hypertrophic, noncompliant right ventricle, cardiac tamponade can develop without echocardiographic signs of right ventricular compression. We prefer to use serial echocardiograms to pre-

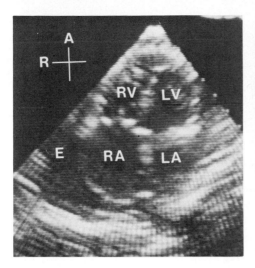 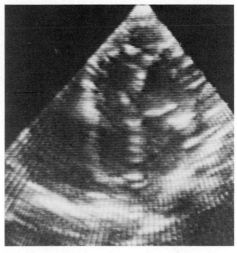

FIG. 13-3. *Apical four-chamber views in systole* (**left**) *and diastole* (**right**) *from a patient with a large pericardial effusion* (E) *following closure of a sinus venosus atrial septal defect. The effusion is seen around the right atrium* (RA), *right ventricle* (RV), *and left ventricle* (LV). *In diastole, the right ventricle is compressed. A, apex; LA, left atrium; R, right.*

dict impending cardiac tamponade rather than a single echocardiographic examination.

Left pleural effusions can sometimes be seen as echo-free spaces posterior to the left ventricle. Unlike pericardial effusions, pleural effusions do not produce a separation between the left ventricular posterior wall and the descending aorta,[5] a factor that may help differentiate pleural and pericardial effusions in the parasternal long-axis view. When a pleural and posterior pericardial effusion are present, the bright echo arising from the posterior pericardium can often be seen separating the two layers of fluid (Fig. 13-6).

PATCHES

Artificial patches used to close atrial and ventricular septal defects and to reconstruct the right ventricular outflow tract give rise to highly reflective echoes. The position of the patch on the atrial or ventricular septum provides information as to the anatomic type of defect that was present. For example, in patients who have undergone closure of an outlet or conotruncal ventricular septal defect, the patch can be seen positioned obliquely from the septum to the anteriorly displaced aorta (Fig. 13-7). Also, in patients who have undergone repair of a complete atrioventricular canal defect, the patch extends from the lower portion of the atrial septum to the upper portion of the ventricular septum in the four-chamber view (Fig. 13-8).

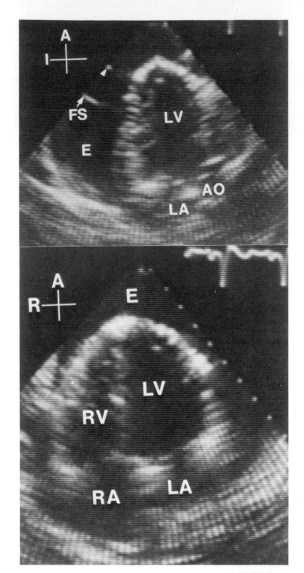

FIG. 13-4. *Apical long-axis view* (**top**) *and apical four-chamber view* (**bottom**) *from a patient with a large pericardial effusion (E) following pulmonary valvotomy. Fibrinous strands (FS) are seen in the pericardial fluid. A, apex; AO, aorta; I, inferior; LA, left atrium; LV, left ventricle; R, right; RA, right atrium; RV, right ventricle.*

FIG. 13-5. *Parasternal short-axis view from a patient with a large pericardial effusion following pulmonary valvotomy. The effusion extends anteriorly around the right ventricle and main pulmonary artery (MPA). A fibrinous strand (arrow) is seen in the effusion. Note the poststenotic dilatation of the left pulmonary artery (LPA). A, anterior; AO, aorta; R, right; RPA, right pulmonary artery.*

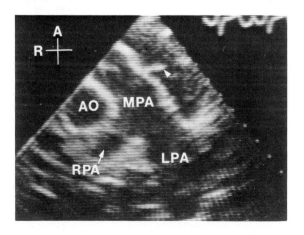

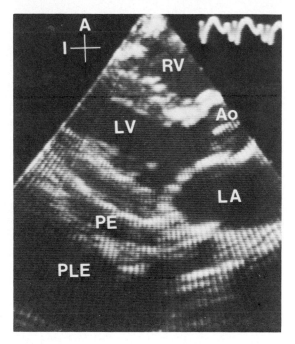

FIG. 13-6. *Parasternal long-axis view from a patient with a small posterior pericardial effusion (PE) and a large left pleural effusion (PLE) following cardiac surgery. The bright echoes arising from the posterior pericardium are seen separating the two effusions. A, anterior; Ao, aorta; I, inferior; LA, left atrium; LV, left ventricle; RV, right ventricle.*

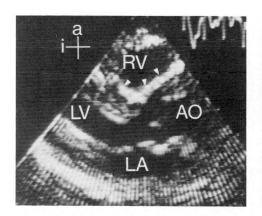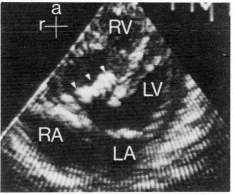

FIG. 13-7. Left. *Parasternal long-axis view from an infant following repair of truncus arteriosus. The patch (arrows) used to close the ventricular septal defect is densely reflective and is positioned obliquely from the septum to the anteriorly-displaced aorta (AO). The position of the patch indicates a previous conotruncal defect. a, anterior; i, inferior; LA, left atrium; LV, left ventricle; RV, right ventricle.* **Right.** *Apical four-chamber view from the same patient. The patch (arrows) is located on the right side of the septum and protrudes into the right ventricle (RV) because of its connection to the overriding aorta. a, apex; LA, left atrium; LV, left ventricle; r, right; RA, right atrium.*

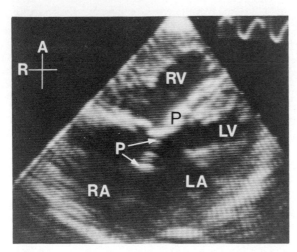

FIG. 13-8. *Apical four-chamber view from a patient following patch repair of a complete atrioventricular canal type A. A pericardial patch (white P) was used to close the primum atrial septal defect (lower portion of atrial septum) and a dacron patch (black P) was used to close the ventricular septal defect (upper portion of the ventricular septum). Note the brighter echoes arising from the dacron patch. The right ventricle (RV) is thickened and apex forming because of previous pulmonary hypertension. A, apex; LA, left atrium; LV, left ventricle; R, right; RA, right atrium.*

In patients who have undergone patch closure of an atrial or ventricular septal defect, residual right-to-left shunting can be detected by peripheral venous contrast echocardiography.[6] In rare instances, the residual defect can be directly visualized on the two-dimensional echocardiogram (Fig. 13-9). In patients who have undergone placement of a patch across a previously narrowed right ventricular outflow tract, aneurysmal dilatation in the area of the patch often can be seen in the parasternal and subcostal short-axis views (Fig. 13-10).

BIOPROSTHETIC VALVES

Because of their low rate of thromboembolism, bioprosthetic valves have been used with increasing frequency in pediatric patients. The most commonly used bioprosthetic valve is the porcine heterograft valve. On the two-dimensional echocardiogram in patients with a heterograft valve, bright echoes are seen arising from the valve stents while very faint echoes arise from the valve leaflets (Figs. 13-11 to 13-13). In order to image the leaflets, high gain and low reject settings are frequently necessary. In order to measure the external stent diameter, which closely approximates the valve size, low gain and high reject settings are necessary.[7] Heterograft valve leaflets that appear thickened and prominent on the two-dimensional echocardiogram should arouse suspicions of a thrombus, vegetation, or valve degeneration (calcific nodules).[8]

Occasionally, direct evidence of bioprosthetic valve malfunction can be seen by two-dimensional echocardiography. For example, the flail leaflet of a heterograft mitral valve can be seen in the left atrium in the long-axis and four-chamber views. Also, dehiscence of a heterograft aortic valve has been

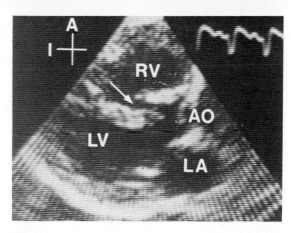

FIG. 13-9. *Parasternal long-axis view from a patient following patch closure of a membranous ventricular septal defect. A residual ventricular septal defect (arrow) caused by disruption of the patch away from the septum is seen. A, anterior; AO, aorta; I, inferior; LA, left atrium; LV, left ventricle; RV, right ventricle.*

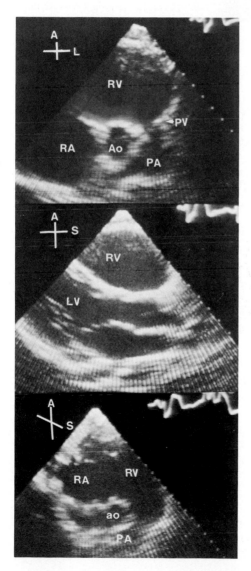

FIG. 13-10. *Parasternal short-axis view* (**top**), *parasternal long-axis view* (**middle**), *and subcostal short-axis view* (**bottom**) *of a patient following repair of tetralogy of Fallot. Aneurysmal dilatation of the right ventricular outflow tract patch can be seen in the short-axis views. A, anterior; Ao, aorta; L, left; LV, left ventricle; PA, pulmonary artery; PV, pulmonary valve; RA, right atrium; RV, right ventricle; S, superior.*

221

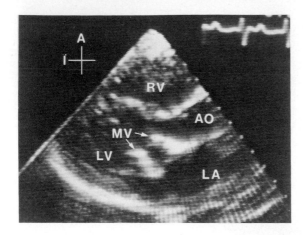

FIG. 13-11. *Parasternal long-axis view from a patient with a heterograft mitral valve (MV). Bright echoes are seen arising from the valve stents, and faint echoes arise from the closed valve leaflets. A, anterior; AO, aorta; I, inferior; LA, left atrium; LV, left ventricle; RV, right ventricle.*

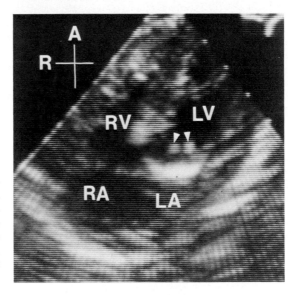

FIG. 13-12. *Apical four-chamber view from a patient with a heterograft mitral valve. Bright echoes can be seen arising from the valve stents (arrows). A, apex; LA, left atrium; LV, left ventricle; R, right; RA, right atrium; RV, right ventricle.*

seen as a separation between the echoes of the valve and the aortic wall.[9] More often, there is indirect evidence on the two-dimensional echocardiogram of heterograft valve stenosis or leakage. For example, left ventricular volume overload can indicate aortic or mitral valve incompetence, and a large left atrium can indicate an obstructive heterograft mitral valve.[7]

CONDUITS

External conduits with heterograft valves are frequently used to connect the right ventricle to the pulmonary arteries in patients with truncus arteriosus, pulmonary atresia, or severe tetralogy of Fallot. As with bioprosthetic valves

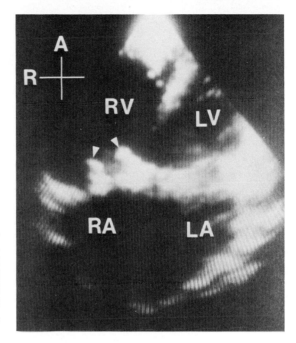

FIG. 13-13. *Apical four-chamber view from a patient with an obstructive heterograft tricuspid valve. The valve stents (arrows) can be seen. The right atrium (RA) is enlarged. A, apex; LA, left atrium; LV, left ventricle; R, right; RV, right ventricle.*

the conduit walls are highly reflective, and the heterograft valve echoes are faint. Low gain and high reject settings are usually necessary to determine the external and internal diameters of the conduit, while high gain and low reject settings are necessary to image the valve leaflets.

The conduit can be imaged best by placing the transducer directly over the area on the precordium that corresponds to the location of the valve ring on the chest x-ray (Fig. 13-14). The transducer can then be oriented in long- and short-axis planes so that the entire conduit can be seen longitudinally or the heterograft valve can be seen in cross section. In many instances, the distal connections of the conduit to the branch pulmonary arteries are difficult to image clearly.

PULMONARY ARTERY BAND

On the two-dimensional echocardiogram, pulmonary artery bands can be seen in the short-axis and suprasternal notch views as a dense white echo across the main pulmonary artery (Fig. 13-15). Often, if the band is effective, the branch pulmonary arteries are small compared with the main pulmonary artery. The suprasternal notch views are especially useful for detecting a band that has migrated to a branch pulmonary artery (Fig. 13-16). In patients who have had a pulmonary artery band removed, an area of residual narrowing frequently can be seen in the area of the pulmonary artery that was previously occupied by the band (Fig. 13-17).

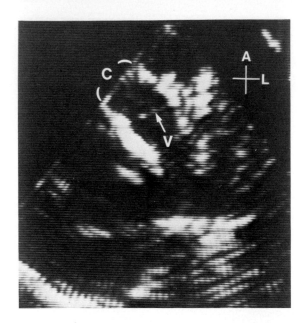

FIG. 13-14. *Parasternal view of a conduit (C). Bright echoes can be seen arising from the conduit walls. Faint echoes can be seen arising from the heterograft valve (V) in the conduit. A, anterior; L, left.*

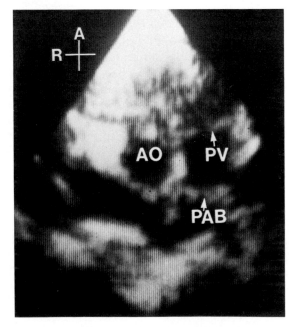

FIG. 13-15. *Parasternal short-axis view from a patient with double outlet right ventricle and a pulmonary artery band (PAB). The bright echoes arising from the band are seen across the main pulmonary artery. A, anterior; AO, aorta; PV, pulmonary valve; R, right.*

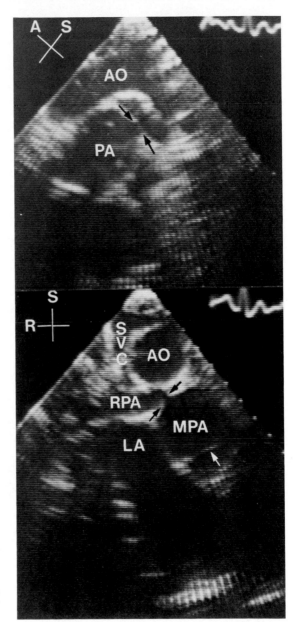

FIG. 13-16. *Suprasternal notch long- (top) and short-(bottom) axis views from a patient with a pulmonary artery band (black arrows). The pulmonary band has migrated distally and is encroaching on the right pulmonary artery (RPA). The pulmonary artery branches are much smaller than the main pulmonary artery (MPA). The white arrow indicates the pulmonary valve. A, anterior; AO, aorta; LA, left atrium; R, right; S, superior; SVC, superior vena cava.*

AORTOPULMONARY SHUNT

We have been able to image an aortopulmonary shunt between the ascending aorta and main pulmonary artery in an infant with pulmonary atresia (Fig. 13-18); however, we have thus far been unable to visualize directly a Blalock–Taussig or Waterston shunt.

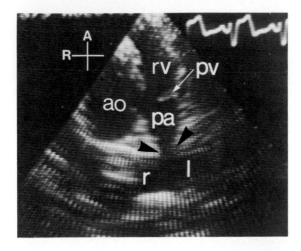

FIG. 13-17. *Parasternal short-axis view from the same patient as in Fig. 13-15 following removal of the pulmonary artery band. An area of residual narrowing (black arrows) is present in the pulmonary artery (pa) at the site of the previous band. A, anterior; ao, aorta; l, left pulmonary artery; pv, pulmonary valve; R, right; r, right pulmonary artery; rv, right ventricle.*

FIG. 13-18. *Parasternal short-axis view from an infant with pulmonary atresia following placement of a 4-mm Gore-tex shunt (white arrow) between the aorta (AO) and main pulmonary artery (PA). Small pulmonary artery branches (black arrows) can be seen. A, anterior; R, right.*

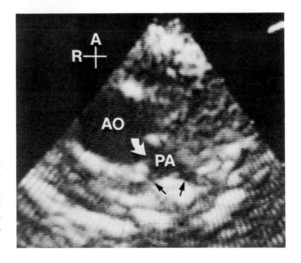

REFERENCES

1. Feigenbaum H, Waldhausen JA, Hyde LP: Ultrasound diagnosis of pericardial effusion. JAMA 191: 711, 1965
2. Horowitz MS, Schultz CS, Stinson EB, Harrison DC, Popp RL: Sensitivity and specificity of echocardiographic diagnosis of pericardial effusion. Circulation 50: 239, 1974
3. Feigenbaum H, Zaky A, Grabhorn LL: Cardiac motion in patients with pericardial effusion: A study using reflected ultrasound. Circulation 34: 611, 1966

4. Schiller NB, Botvinick EH: Right ventricular compression as a sign of cardiac tamponade. An analysis of echocardiographic ventricular dimensions and their clinical implications. Circulation 56: 774, 1977

5. Haaz WS, Mintz GS, Kotler MN, Parry WR: Two-dimensional echocardiographic recognition of the descending thoracic aorta: Value in differentiating pericardial from pleural effusions. Am J Cardiol 45: 401, 1980

6. Valdes-Cruz LM, Pieroni DR, Roland J-MA, Shematek JP: Recognition of residual postoperative shunts by contrast echocardiographic techniques. Circulation 55: 148, 1977

7. Feigenbaum H: Echocardiography. Philadelphia, Lea and Febiger, 1981, pp. 298–315

8. Alam M, Madrazo AC, Magilligan DJ, Goldstein S: M-mode and two-dimensional echocardiographic features of porcine valve dysfunction. Am J Cardiol 43: 502, 1979

9. Schapira JN, Martin RP, Fowles RE, Rakowski H, Stinson EB, French JW, Shumway NE, Popp RL: Two-dimensional echocardiographic assessment of patients with bioprosthetic valves. Am J Cardiol 43: 510, 1979

CHAPTER 14

A Segmental Approach to the Diagnosis of Cardiac Situs and Malpositions

Although M-mode echocardiography has been useful in evaluating cardiac malpositions, the technique is limited by its inability to define spatial relations. Deduction of structure positions is made solely by the examiner.[1-3] Two-dimensional echocardiography, by virtue of its ability to display structures spatially, offers substantial advantages over M-mode echocardiography for the evaluation of complex congenital cardiac malformations.

The two-dimensional echocardiogram can be combined with simultaneous M-mode echocardiography and contrast echocardiography for structure validation.[4] The echocardiogram can be performed independently of other noninvasive assessments such as the clinical examination, chest roentgenogram, and electrocardiogram; but a more rapid and complete evaluation can be achieved when all these modalities are combined.

A sequential approach to the evaluation of cardiac malpositions can be used. In this approach, the cardiac situs is first determined. Then, the atrioventricular connections are established and the ventricular morphology is defined. Finally, the ventriculoarterial connections and relations are established. There are two ways in which this information can be obtained (Table 14-1). The first method is to perform a routine echocardiographic examination, gleaning information from each plane as it is obtained. The second method is to examine each of the segmental areas of the heart in sequence using multiple planes. The latter approach is time consuming because of the repetition of views used to evaluate each segment. The former approach is more desirable as it uses a step-by-step integration of the information derived from each of the planes as they are performed in sequence in the routine examination (see Chapter 3). A routine sequence ensures that information is not missed.

TABLE 14-1. SEGMENTAL ANALYSIS OF THE HEART BY TWO-DIMENSIONAL ECHOCARDIOGRAPHY

	Plane
ATRIAL SITUS	
Connection of superior and inferior venae cavae with anatomic right atrium	Subcostal long- and short-axis Contrast echocardiography Suprasternal short-axis
Connection of pulmonary veins with anatomic left atrium	Apical four-chamber Subcostal four-chamber
Inference from pulmonary artery anatomy and bronchial relationships	Suprasternal long- and short-axis
Inference from aorta and inferior vena cava positions	Subcostal long- and short-axis
VENTRICULAR MORPHOLOGY	
Definition of anatomic left ventricle	
Two papillary muscles	Parasternal short-axis
"Fish-mouth" valve (mitral valve)	Parasternal short-axis
Atrioventricular valve further from cardiac apex	Apical four-chamber
Definition of anatomic right ventricle	
Moderator band	Apical four-chamber
Coarse trabecular pattern equals right ventricle	Apical and subcostal four-chamber
Atrioventricular valve closer to cardiac apex	Apical four-chamber
ATRIOVENTRICULAR CONNECTIONS	
Concordant or discordant, double inlet ventricle, absent right or left connections, straddling atrioventricular valve	Apical four-chamber Subcostal four-chamber
VENTRICULOARTERIAL CONNECTIONS	
Presence of one or two semilunar valves	Parasternal long- and short-axis
Vessel that bifurcates equals pulmonary artery	Parasternal short-axis Subcostal short-axis
Relationship of semilunar valves to ventricular septum and ventricles	Parasternal long- and short-axis
POSITION OF CARDIAC APEX	
Dextrocardia, Mesocardia, Levocardia	Apical four-chamber Subcostal four-chamber
AORTIC ARCH	
Right- or left-sided arch Detection of thoracic aorta	Suprasternal long-axis Subcostal long-axis Apical long-axis Parasternal short-axis

In cardiac malpositions, terminology is an unsettled issue. We favor a descriptive approach that could be applied to any of the existing systems of nomenclature.[5-7]

THE PARASTERNAL LONG-AXIS PLANE

In cardiac malpositions, the plane for obtaining the parasternal long-axis view may be different. First, an attempt should be made to obtain the standard parasternal long-axis view with the plane oriented between the left hip and right shoulder. If the parasternal long-axis view cannot be obtained in this plane, then several other transducer positions should be attempted to image the long-axis view. For example, the transducer can be placed in the right chest in a plane parallel to the standard long-axis plane. This technique is useful for obtaining a long-axis view in patients with dextroposition (i.e., heart shifted to the right due to pulmonary disease). In patients with situs inversus and dextrocardia, the long-axis view is obtained from the right side of the sternum in a plane oriented between the right hip and left shoulder (the mirror image of the standard long-axis plane). In transposition of the great arteries, the long-axis plane is oriented slightly more vertically than usual because the pulmonary artery is positioned to the left of the aorta's normal position. When dextrocardia is present, it is helpful to examine the patient in a right lateral decubitus position.

In malpositions in which the heart is retrosternal or the ventricles and great vessels have a complex arrangement, it may not be possible to obtain a recognizable long-axis view. These complex spatial arrangements may lead to unusual appearances of the cardiac chambers in certain views. For example, in l-transposition with ventricular inversion, the ventricular septum can lie perpendicular to the chest wall and parallel to the long-axis plane. Therefore, the long-axis view can be obtained without imaging the ventricular septum, and the erroneous impression of a univentricular heart can be perceived. The use of other views and contrast echocardiography can help eliminate this problem.

Several features of the parasternal long-axis plane are helpful in determining chamber identification and ventriculoarterial connections. The continuity of the posterior great vessel and the anterior mitral valve leaflet (see Fig. 3-4) helps define the left ventricle. This continuity is lost in double outlet right ventricle (see Fig. 9-17). Also, the continuity between the ventricular septum and the posterior great vessel, which is disturbed in tetralogy of Fallot (see Fig. 9-1), truncus arteriosus (see Fig. 9-10), and double outlet right ventricle, can be assessed in the long-axis view. In transposition of the great arteries, the parallel spatial relations of the great arteries as they exit the heart can be identified (see Figs. 10-5 to 10-7). In addition, the posterior sweep of the posterior great vessel helps define the pulmonary artery. In single ventricle, the connections between the ventricle, the outflow chamber, and the great vessels can often be determined in the long-axis plane (see Fig. 12-11).

THE PARASTERNAL SHORT-AXIS PLANE

The parasternal short-axis plane provides important information concerning the laterality of structures, the morphology of the ventricles and the atrioventricular valves, and the ventriculoarterial connections. Regardless of where on the precordium the short-axis is obtained, the examiner should orient the index mark toward the patient's left side so as not to disturb the right–left orientation on the videoscreen. As with the normal heart, the transducer should be rotated approximately 90 degrees clockwise from the long-axis plane to obtain the short-axis image. With malpositions, this plane can be altered depending on the orientation of the major axis of the heart. As with the parasternal long-axis plane in malposition, when the heart is lying behind the sternum, it may not be possible to obtain complete evaluation from this plane.

In situs inversus with dextrocardia, the short-axis plane is the mirror image of the standard short-axis plane and is oriented between the right shoulder and left hip (Fig. 14-1). There is reversal of the direction of the right ventricular outflow tract and pulmonary artery as they course around the aortic root. Anomalies of situs can be associated with more complex pathology, such as in Figure 14-2 where the patient also had tetralogy of Fallot.

The short-axis view at the base of the heart is especially useful for defining ventriculoarterial connections such as double outlet right ventricle, truncus arteriosus, or transposition of the great vessels (see Chapters 9 and 10).

In transposition, the great vessels are seen as "double circles" in the short-axis view (see Chapter 10). With cranial angulation of the transducer, the posterior pulmonary artery can be seen bifurcating into its two branches (Fig. 14-3). This view defines the ventriculoarterial connection (transposition) as well as the spatial relations of the two great arteries.

When there is dextroposition due to pulmonary disease, diaphragmatic hernia, or other causes that result in a right mediastinal shift, the short-axis

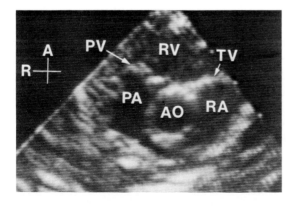

FIG. 14-1. *Parasternal short-axis view obtained from the right parasternal area in a patient with dextrocardia and situs inversus. Note that the right atrium (RA) and tricuspid valve (TV) are on the left, and the pulmonary valve (PV) and pulmonary arteries (PA) are on the right. The aorta (AO) is a circular structure in the center of the image. The great vessels form a "circle-sausage" pattern in the mirror image of the normal relationships, indicating situs inversus with concordant ventriculoarterial connections. A, anterior; R, right; RV, right ventricle.*

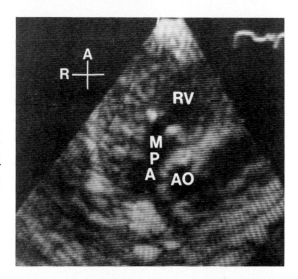

FIG. 14-2. *Parasternal short-axis plane at the level of the great vessels from a patient with situs inversus, dextrocardia, and tetralogy of Fallot. The bifurcation of the main pulmonary artery (MPA) into the right and left branches can be identified to the right of the aorta (AO). The stenotic pulmonary valve can be identified between the MPA and right ventricle (RV). A, anterior; R, right.*

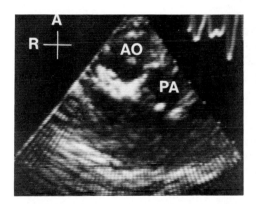
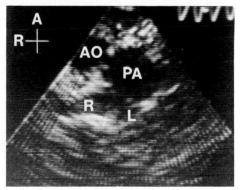

FIG. 14-3. *Parasternal short-axis view at the level of the great vessels from a patient with situs inversus, d-loop, and d-transposition of the great arteries. The aorta (AO) is anterior and to the right of the pulmonary artery (PA). Slight cranial angulation (right) defines the right (R) and left (L) pulmonary artery branches, confirming that the posterior vessel is the pulmonary artery. A, anterior; R, right.*

view of the great vessels is obtained from the right precordium in a plane parallel to the normal short-axis view. The short-axis view from this location has a normal right–left orientation.

The short-axis view through the ventricles shows certain anatomic features that help distinguish the right from the left ventricle. The two papillary muscles of the left ventricle are readily defined. In addition, the mitral valve is a bicommissural valve that has a characteristic "fish-mouth" appearance. These two features characterize the left ventricle whether it is found on the left or right of the right ventricle (Fig. 14-4).

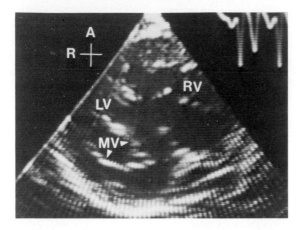

FIG. 14-4. *A parasternal short-axis plane at the level of the ventricles obtained from the right precordium of a patient with dextrocardia, situs inversus, and tetralogy of Fallot. The "fish-mouth" mitral valve (MV) can be seen in the circular left ventricle (LV). The left ventricle is to the right and posterior of the right ventricle (RV). The dropout of echoes from the ventricular septum is a ventricular septal defect. A, anterior; R, right.*

APICAL FOUR-CHAMBER PLANE

To obtain the apical four-chamber view, the cardiac apex should be located by palpation. When it is difficult to palpate the cardiac apex, the transducer can be moved around in the region where the apex is suspected to be until a representative image is obtained. When properly obtained, the image should have the cardiac apex in the apex of the fan. In situs inversus with dextrocardia, the transducer is positioned in a plane that is the mirror image of the standard four-chamber plane.

The transducer position used to obtain the apical views defines whether there is levocardia with the apex pointing to the left, mesocardia with the apex pointing to the midline (Fig. 14-5), or dextrocardia (Fig. 14-6) with the apex

FIG. 14-5. *Subcostal four-chamber view from a patient with mesocardia. The right ventricle (RV) is right sided and the left ventricle (LV) is left sided. A ventricular septal defect can be seen in the posterior portion of the ventricular septum. Note that the cardiac apex is pointing toward the apex of the fan, indicating mesocardia. The liver and diaphragm are anterior to the heart. A, anterior; R, right.*

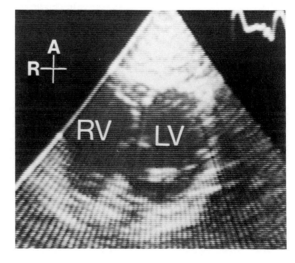

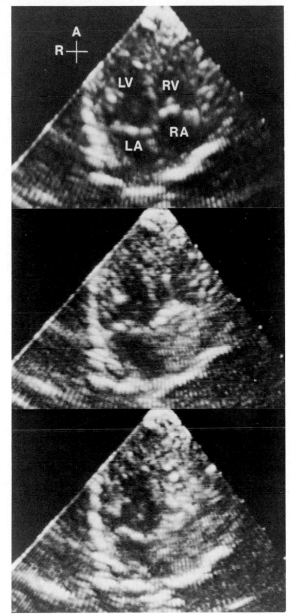

FIG. 14-6. Top. *An apical four-chamber view from an infant with situs inversus and dextrocardia. This view was obtained by applying the transducer below the right nipple. The right ventricle (RV) and right atrium (RA) are left-sided structures. The left atrium (LA) and left ventricle (LV) are right-sided structures. The right-sided atrioventricular valve (mitral valve) is further from the cardiac apex than the left-sided atrioventricular valve. Also, the pulmonary veins are draining to the right-sided anatomic left atrium. A, apex; R, right.* **Middle and Bottom.** *A contrast injection was made into a right arm vein. The contrast echoes fill the left-sided anatomic right atrium and then flow into the left-sided anatomic right ventricle. Thus, this patient has situs inversus, l-loop (anatomic right ventricle on the left), and normally related great vessels.*

pointing towards the right. This contribution of the two-dimensional echocardiogram is useful because the frontal chest film may not show the precise position of the cardiac apex.

For the apical four-chamber view, the transducer index mark should remain oriented toward the patient's left side. There are characteristic anatomic features of the left ventricle, the right ventricle, the left atrium, and the right atrium (see Chapter 3), and identification of these features in the four-chamber view is helpful for defining the atrioventricular connections and for inferring the ventriculoarterial connections. The following examples illustrate the use of this plane.

The apical four-chamber view in Figure 14-6 is of a newborn infant with dextrocardia. The image was obtained from the fourth right intercostal space in the midclavicular line, and it confirmed the presence of dextrocardia with the cardiac apex pointing towards the right. The atrioventricular valve on the left is closer to the cardiac apex than that on the right, indicating that the left-sided ventricle is an anatomic right ventricle. On the right side, the mitral valve is located further from the cardiac apex. Also, in the parasternal short-axis view, the right-sided ventricle had features of an anatomic left ventricle (two papillary muscles). The pulmonary veins are seen draining to the right-sided atrium, suggesting that this atrium is the anatomic left atrium. The contrast echocardiogram performed from an arm vein demonstrates that the systemic veins drained to the left-sided anatomic right atrium. The left atrium connects to the anatomic left ventricle, and the right atrium connects to the anatomic right ventricle. The atrioventricular connections are normal, and the four chambers are positioned in a mirror image of normal. The final diagnosis is situs inversus with dextrocardia, l-loop (anatomic right ventricle on the left), and normally related great vessels.

The apical four-chamber views of the next patient (Figs. 14-7 and 14-8) were obtained from the fifth left intercostal space at the midclavicular line, indicating levocardia. The pulmonary veins enter the left-sided atrium, indi-

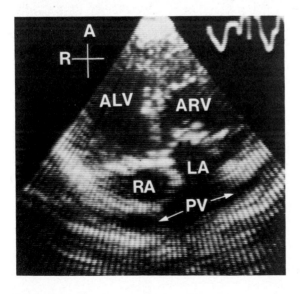

FIG. 14-7. *An apical four-chamber view from the left precordium in the usual position. The pulmonary veins (PV) are seen draining into the left-sided left atrium (LA), indicating situs solitus. The left-sided atrioventricular valve lies closer to the cardiac apex, and a prominent moderator band is present in the left-sided ventricle. These features define the left-sided ventricle as an anatomic right ventricle (ARV). The anatomic left ventricle (ALV) has a smooth outline and an atrioventricular valve further from the cardiac apex. This patient has discordant atrioventricular connections and a diagnosis of situs solitus, l-loop (anatomic right ventricle on the left), and l-transposition. A, anterior; R, right; RA, right atrium.*

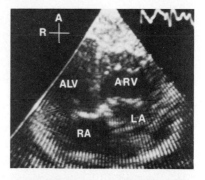

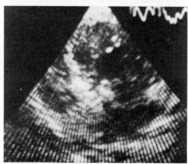

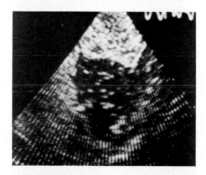

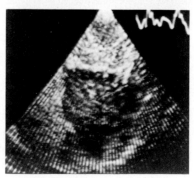

FIG. 14-8. *Contrast echocardiogram into a right arm vein in the same patient as in Fig. 14-7.* **Top.** *Apical four-chamber view prior to contrast injection. A, apex; ALV, anatomic left ventricle; ARV, anatomic right ventricle; LA, left atrium; R, right; RA, right atrium.* **Second.** *Contrast echoes fill the right-sided atrium, confirming the diagnosis of situs solitus.* **Third and Fourth frames.** *A small right-to-left ventricular shunt is seen.*

cating that this is the anatomic left atrium (Fig. 14-7). A contrast injection (Fig. 14-8) fills the right-sided atrium, indicating that this is the anatomic right atrium and that there is normal cardiac situs. A small right-to-left ventricular shunt is present. Inspection of the right-sided ventricle shows that it is an anatomic left ventricle because it is smooth walled and has an atrioventricular valve that is further from the apex. The left-sided ventricle is an anatomic right ventricle because it has coarse trabeculations in its apex, a prominent moderator band, and an atrioventricular valve that is situated closer to the cardiac apex. The atrioventricular connections are, therefore, discordant. In the parasternal short-axis view, there was l-transposition of the great vessels. The patient's diagnosis is situs solitus, l-loop (anatomic right ventricle on the left), l-transposition, and ventricular septal defect.

The apical four-chamber view in Figure 14-9 was obtained from the fifth right intercostal space, indicating dextrocardia. A contrast injection fills the left-sided atrium, indicating that it is an anatomic right atrium and that there is situs inversus. The anatomic right ventricle, with its moderator band and atrioventricular valve closer to the cardiac apex, is seen on the right side. The left-sided ventricle is smooth walled and has an atrioventricular valve further from the apex, defining it as an anatomic left ventricle. In the parasternal short-axis view, the great vessels were d-transposed. This patient's final diagnosis is situs inversus with dextrocardia, d-loop (anatomic right ventricle on the right), d-transposition, and ventricular septal defect.

All of the anatomic features described above are not usually present in every patient's apical four-chamber view. For example in the patient with situs inversus shown in Figure 14-10 the right-sided ventricle has trabeculations in its apex, and the left-sided ventricle is smooth walled. However, the spatial relations of the right and left atrioventricular valves indicate that the right-sided valve is a mitral valve and the left-sided valve is a tricuspid valve. The trabecular patterns of the ventricles are poorly defined in this individual because of the inability to image the apical four-chamber view properly. In evaluating cardiac malpositions, it is important to integrate all the information from all the planes.

In situs ambiguus, the definition of atrial anatomy can be difficult. The patient in Figure 14-11 has polysplenia (left isomerism) and an endocardial cushion defect. There are no anatomic features in this view to distinguish an anatomic right atrium or an anatomic left atrium. A contrast injection into a left arm vein shows that there is a left superior vena cava draining directly to the left-sided atrium. A contrast injection into a right arm vein shows that there is a right superior vena cava draining to the right-sided atrium. Patients with situs ambiguus frequently have bilateral superior venae cavae draining directly to both atria and anomalous pulmonary venous connections, making it impossible to define atrial situs.

The apical four-chamber view is valuable for defining absence of the left or right atrioventricular connection (see Fig. 12-13) and double inlet ventricle (see Fig. 12-10).

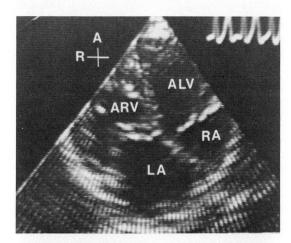

FIG. 14-9. Top. *Apical four-chamber view obtained from the area of the right nipple. The left-sided ventricle is smooth walled and has an atrioventricular valve further from the cardiac apex, indicating that it is the anatomic left ventricle (ALV). The right-sided ventricle has a prominent moderator band and an atrioventricular valve closer to the cardiac apex, indicating that it is an anatomic right ventricle (ARV). The atrial anatomy cannot be defined because the pulmonary veins cannot be clearly seen. A, anterior; R, right; LA, left atrium; RA, right atrium.* **Middle.** *A contrast injection into an arm vein fills the left-sided atrium and ventricle, confirming that the anatomic right atrium is left-sided and that there is situs inversus.* **Bottom.** *A few microcavitations are observed in the anatomic right ventricle, indicating a small right-to-left ventricular shunt. The patient's diagnosis is situs inversus, d-loop (anatomic right ventricle on the the right), d-transposition, and ventricular septal defect.*

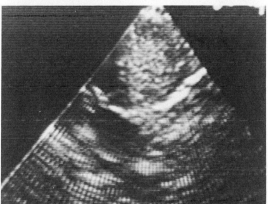

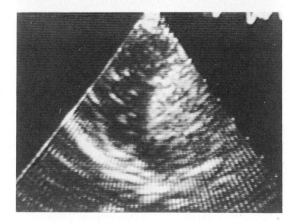

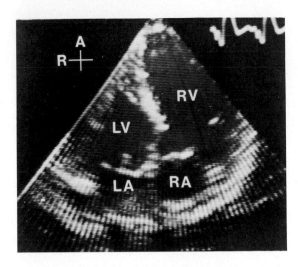

FIG. 14-10. *An apical four-chamber plane from a patient with situs inversus. This particular plane was not obtained precisely from the cardiac apex. The right ventricle (RV) appears smooth walled, and the left ventricle (LV) appears to have coarse echoes in its apex. These echoes arise from the papillary muscles of the left ventricle. The right-sided atrioventricular valve is further from the cardiac apex and is, therefore, the mitral valve. The pulmonary veins are seen entering the right-sided atrium, defining this as an anatomic left atrium (LA). A, apex; R, right; RA, right atrium.*

THE SUBCOSTAL PLANES

The subcostal long-axis plane is useful for defining the aortic and inferior vena caval spatial relations. In addition, the inferior vena cava can be traced to its connection with the anatomic right atrium. Interruption of the inferior vena cava is frequently associated with polysplenia (left isomerism) and can be detected in the subcostal long-axis view (Fig. 14-12).[6,8] The diagnosis of interruption of the inferior vena cava can only be made after an extensive search in the long-axis plane for the lower inferior vena cava. The subcostal short-axis view through the vessels in the abdomen is helpful in establishing their spatial relations. In situs inversus, the aorta is to the right and posterior of the inferior vena cava (Fig. 14-13).

The subcostal four-chamber view, like the apical four-chamber view, allows definition of atrial anatomy, atrioventricular connections, ventricular morphology, and ventriculoarterial connections. The subcostal four-chamber view provides visual display of the position of the cardiac apex. In mesocardia, for example, the apex points toward the transducer (Fig. 14-6). Imaging the apex in mesocardia can produce circular ventricular outlines lying side by side.

In the subcostal short-axis view at the base of the heart, the ventriculoarterial connections can be defined (see Fig. 12-15). In addition, the inferior vena cava–right atrial junction and the Eustachian valve help identify the anatomic right atrium. Pulmonary veins can be traced to the anatomic left atrium from this view as well.[9,10]

THE SUPRASTERNAL PLANES

The suprasternal long-axis view defines the ascending, transverse, and descending aorta. The usual plane runs from the right nipple to the left scapular tip. When the aortic arch is right sided, the examiner has to rotate the plane

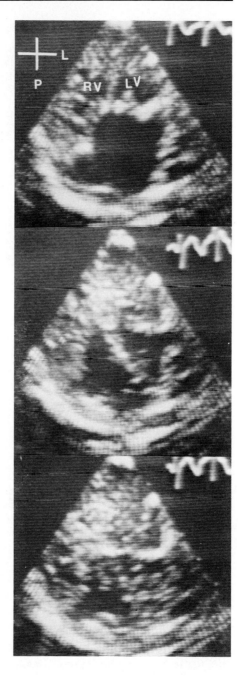

FIG. 14-11. Top. *Apical four-chamber plane obtained from below the left nipple. There are no particular anatomic features to distinguish the right and left atria. L, left; LV, left ventricle; P, posterior; RV, right ventricle.* **Middle.** *A contrast echocardiogram was made from a left arm vein. The contrast bolus appears initially in the left-sided atrium and then flows through both atrioventricular valves (***Bottom***). This finding suggests situs ambiguus.*

counterclockwise until the entire aortic arch can be imaged.[11] The degree of rotation can range between 30 and 90 degrees. The plane in which the aortic arch is imaged should be noted because it cannot be determined by viewing the recorded image. Occasionally the suprasternal long-axis view of the aortic arch can be obtained from the infraclavicular area. This frequently occurs in

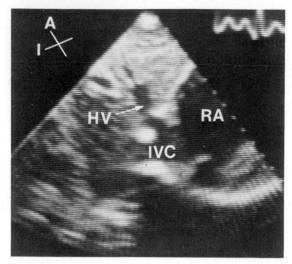

FIG. 14-12. *Subcostal long-axis plane demonstrating the connections between the hepatic vein (HV), inferior vena cava (IVC), and right atrium (RA) in a patient with polysplenia and interrupted inferior vena cava. No continuity between the upper inferior vena cava and any other venous structure can be demonstrated below the level of the hepatic veins. A, anterior; I, inferior.*

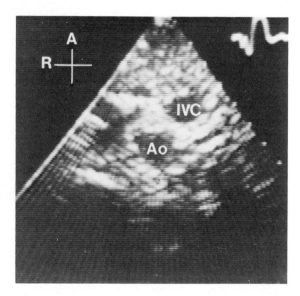

FIG. 14-13. *A subcostal short-axis plane in a patient with situs inversus, demonstrating the inferior vena cava (IVC) and aorta (Ao) in cross section. The inferior vena cava is anterior and to the left of the aorta. A, anterior; R, right.*

situs solitus, l-loop, l-transposition where the aortic arch can be imaged in the left infraclavicular area and in *situs inversus,* d-loop, d-transposition where the aortic arch can be imaged in the right infraclavicular area (see Fig. 10-24).

In the suprasternal long-axis plane the bronchial–pulmonary artery relationships help define the body situs.[12,13] The right pulmonary artery is circular and the right mainstem bronchus, an eparterial bronchus, intercedes between the pulmonary artery and the aortic arch.[11] When the transducer is oriented toward the left from the suprasternal long-axis view, the pulmonary artery appears as a comma-shaped structure. The circular portion is the main pulmonary artery, and the tail is the left pulmonary artery (see Fig. 3-27). No bronchial tissue intercedes between the left pulmonary artery and the aorta because the left bronchus is a hyparterial structure. In conditions with abnormal situs, diminished pulmonary blood flow, and distortion of the pulmonary artery anatomy, these bronchial-pulmonary artery relations are less helpful for defining the atrial situs.

In the suprasternal short-axis plane, the spatial position of the superior vena cava can be established and its connection to the anatomic right atrium defined. This connection can be confirmed by contrast echocardiography. Bilateral superior venae cavae, especially common in patients with situs ambiguus, can be identified from the suprasternal short-axis view (Fig. 14-14). In the normal patient, the right pulmonary artery in the suprasternal short-axis plane can be seen from its junction with the main pulmonary artery to its branches in the right lung. In situs inversus the longitudinal course of the right pulmonary artery from the main pulmonary artery to the right hilum is reversed. Also, the innominate veins join to form the superior vena cava on the left side of the aorta (Fig. 14-15).

INTEGRATION OF THE SEGMENTS

Table 14-1 is a guide to the integration of the cardiac segments. Two-dimensional echocardiography should not be used alone to assess cardiac malpositions but should be integrated with the clinical, electrocardiographic, and radiologic information to give as accurate a diagnosis as possible.

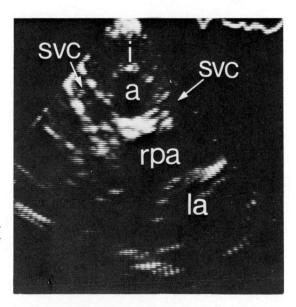

FIG. 14-14. *Suprasternal short-axis view from a patient with situs ambiguus and bilateral superior venae cavae (svc). Note the innominate vein joining the venae cavae. a, aorta; la, left atrium; rpa, right pulmonary artery.*

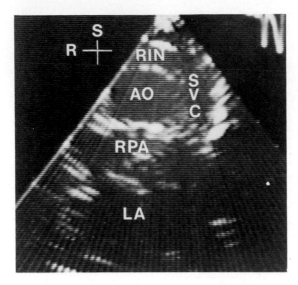

FIG. 14-15. *Suprasternal short-axis plane from a patient with situs inversus. The right innominate vein (RIN) can be seen joining the superior vena cava (SVC) to the left of the aorta (AO). The pulmonary artery can be identified posterior to the aorta. The right pulmonary artery (RPA) arises from the main pulmonary artery on the right and passes toward the left. The left atrium (LA) can be observed posterior to the pulmonary artery. R, right; S, superior.*

REFERENCES

1. Solinger R, Elbl F, Minhas K: Deductive echocardiographic analysis in infants with congenital heart disease. Circulation 50: 1072, 1974

2. Meyer RA, Schwartz DC, Covitz W, Kaplan S: Echocardiographic assessment of cardiac malposition. Am J Cardiol 33: 896, 1974

3. Mortera C, Hunter S, Terry G, Tynan M: Echocardiography of primitive ventricle. Br Heart J 39: 847, 1977

4. Silverman NH, Snider AR, Colo J: A segmental approach to the diagnosis of congenital heart disease: The usefulness of two-dimensional echocardiography. In Echocardiography, S Hunter, R Hall, eds. Edinburgh, Churchill-Livingston, 1981

5. Van Praagh R, Weinberg PW, Van Praagh S: Malpositions of the heart. In Heart Disease in Infants, Children, and Adolescents, AJ Moss, FH Adams, GC Emmanouilides, eds. Baltimore, Williams & Wilkins, 1977

6. Stanger P, Rudolph AM, Edwards JE: Cardiac malpositions: An overview based on a study of sixty-five necropsy specimens. Circulation 52: 159, 1977

7. Tynan MJ, Becker AE, Macartney FJ, Quero-Jimenez M, Shinebourne EA, Anderson RH: Nomenclature and classification of congenital heart disease. Br Heart J 41: 554, 1979

8. Rose V, Izukawa T, Moes CAF: Syndromes of asplenia and polysplenia. Br Heart J 37: 840, 1975

9. Bierman FZ, Williams RG: Subxyphoid two-dimensional imaging of the interatrial septum in infants and neonates with congenital heart disease. Circulation 60: 80, 1979

10. Lange LW, Sahn DJ, Allen HD, Goldberg SJ: Subxyphoid cross-sectional echocardiography in infants and children with congenital heart disease. Circulation 59: 513, 1979

11. Snider AR, Silverman NH: Suprasternal notch echocardiography: A two-dimen-

sional technique for evaluating congenital heart disease. Circulation 63: 165, 1981

12. Van Mierop LHS, Eisen S, Schiebler GL: The radiologic appearance of the tracheobronchial tree as an indicator of visceral situs. Am J Cardiol 26: 432, 1970

13. Partridge JB, Scott O, Deverall PB, Macartney FJ: Visualization and measurement of the main bronchi by tomography as an objective indicator of thoracic situs in congenital heart disease. Circulation 51: 188, 1975

CHAPTER 15

The Assessment of Chamber Size and Ventricular Function

An important emerging function of two-dimensional echocardiography is its use for evaluating cardiac chamber size and function. Because the heart chambers can be viewed from several planes it is possible to obtain a three-dimensional reconstruction of them. Measurement of ejection fraction by two-dimensional echocardiography is more accurate than by M-mode echocardiography because of the former's ability to view contraction of larger areas of the heart. The advantage of the echocardiographic technique over cineangiography seems to be that it has greater accessibility, it is not influenced by contrast injections, and it provides multiple cardiac cycles for analysis.

TECHNICAL CONSIDERATIONS FOR ANALYZING CARDIAC CHAMBER SIZE BY TWO-DIMENSIONAL ECHOCARDIOGRAPHY

Resolution

Ultrasound has technical limitations that must be considered when estimating volume by two-dimensional echocardiography. It is obvious that the better the resolution of the instrument the more accurately the observer will be able to trace the endocardial outline. Axial resolution is better than lateral resolution and is usually less than 1.5 mm. Lateral resolution varies considerably within the field and is better toward the center of the sector scan. In order to make use of the best resolution of the echocardiographic system the chamber that is to be evaluated should be placed as close as possible to the center of the sector.

Gain Settings

It has been shown that the size of the image may vary in proportion to the magnitude of the gain on the instrument.[1-3] With high gain settings experiments have shown that the targets appear closer to one another. Therefore, in order to record the endocardium of a chamber for volume analysis the gains should be adjusted to be at the lowest setting consistent with satisfactory resolution.

Calibration

Most current commercial systems provide only a depth calibration. Unfortunately, as no breadth calibration is available, changes in the adjustments on the videomonitor system may produce significant changes in the vertical and horizontal representation of the image. To ensure that these settings are as true as possible, a protractor should be used to measure the angle of the fan on the videomonitor. The height and breadth of the videomonitor are then adjusted to yield the appropriate angle consistent with the manufacturer's specifications. Subsequently, measurements should be made using a test block standard to ensure appropriate instrument calibration.

Tracing of the Image

Tracing the outline of the chamber directly from a videomonitor rather than from a photographic print diminishes the manual errors, because the minor inaccuracies related to the tracings are magnified by using a small format.

We favor some direct tracing of the endocardial outline from a frozen frame of a video image performed with a light pen. A system using a light pen allows inspection of the accuracy of the tracing before analysis, unlike some systems where the traced outline cannot be inspected for accuracy. The light pen system eliminates the significant problem of parallax that can be produced by tracing on a clear plastic overlay directly from the video monitor.

Precise display of the entire endocardium generally is not possible on any one frame. Areas of dropout related to technical factors or true anatomic defects require that extrapolation be made between points. In these circumstances the outline can be completed by drawing a straight line between the adjacent endocardial echoes, after referring to preceding and succeeding beats. In order to ensure accuracy each area should be calculated at least three times. In this manner the observer can evaluate the accuracy of the tracing by noting the variability and can derive an average measurement.

Computers

Volume analysis should be performed using a computer. The area of the chamber may be rapidly planimetered, its length obtained, and the information stored in the computer memory bank. By having such a facility a variety of algorithms may be programmed into the computer to calculate the volume of any particular chamber. To date there are only a limited number of commercially available systems that have either preprogrammed algorithms or have the flexibility of allowing the users to write their own program for volume calculation. Computer-aided recognition of outline has been established and may be adapted in the near future for two-dimensional echocardiography to allow automated assessment of chamber volume. As it currently requires approximately 30 minutes to perform a volume estimation, a system such as automated edge detection, which diminishes this time considerably, will simplify the estimation of ventricular volumes and cardiac function.

Timing of End-Diastole and End-Systole

The selection of which frame to analyze may be made by reference to another physiological event. The electrocardiogram is the most widely used physiologic reference. Some ultrasound instruments present, in addition, a second physiologic variable such as a pulse or a phonocardiogram on the video monitor. The high frequency of the heart sounds recorded by phonocardiography makes this a more desirable means of defining cardiac events for volume analysis with regard to timing of end-systole.

LEFT VENTRICULAR VOLUME DETERMINATION AND FUNCTION

Recent studies have shown that left ventricular volume and ejection fraction can be calculated accurately by two-dimensional echocardiography from infancy to adulthood.[4-13] Two-dimensional echocardiography appears to be more accurate than M-mode echocardiography for determining these indices of left ventricular function. There are several models that can be used to calculate left ventricular volume (Fig. 15-1). Single-plane estimates of ventricular volume have been compared with ventricular volume calculated by angiography, using the ventricular outline traced from the apical long-axis or apical four-chamber planes. Most studies use a combination of images generated from different planes to determine volume. To this end several algorithms have been used (Fig. 15-1).

For children we have used the apical four-chamber and apical long-axis planes (Figs. 15-2 and 15-3). This choice was based on the reasoning that, as with angiography, both planes are orthogonal and share a common long axis that makes it suitable for analysis by Simpson's rule and biplane area-length methods. The areas of the ventricles were traced using a light pen interfaced with a microprocessor that was programmed to calculate the area, and with the long length of the ventricle taken to be between the apex and the closed mitral valve leaflets.[10] For the apical four-chamber view the outline is traced on the endocardial surface of the apex, the ventricular septal endocardium, and through the plane of the opposed mitral valve leaflets. The outline is com-

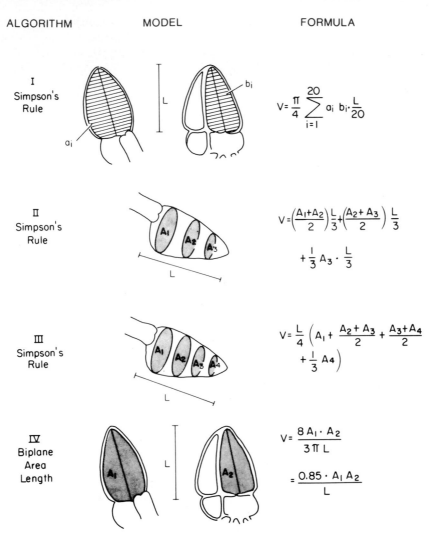

ALGORITHM   MODEL   FORMULA

I
Simpson's
Rule

$$V = \frac{\pi}{4} \sum_{i=1}^{20} a_i \, b_i \cdot \frac{L}{20}$$

II
Simpson's
Rule

$$V = \left(\frac{A_1 + A_2}{2}\right) \frac{L}{3} + \left(\frac{A_2 + A_3}{2}\right) \frac{L}{3}$$
$$+ \frac{1}{3} A_3 \cdot \frac{L}{3}$$

III
Simpson's
Rule

$$V = \frac{L}{4} \left(A_1 + \frac{A_2 + A_3}{2} + \frac{A_3 + A_4}{2} \right.$$
$$\left. + \frac{1}{3} A_4 \right)$$

IV
Biplane
Area
Length

$$V = \frac{8 \, A_1 \cdot A_2}{3 \pi L}$$
$$= \frac{0.85 \cdot A_1 \, A_2}{L}$$

FIG. 15-1. *A demonstration of various biplane and single plane methods used to cal-culate chamber volume.* **I.** *Simpson's rule method based on orthogonal planes from the apical long-axis and apical four-chamber plane. The calculation is based on the sum-mation of areas from diameters* a_i *and* b_i *of 20 equal cylinders obtained by dividing the left ventricular longest length* (L) *into 20 equal sections.* **II.** *Simpson's rule using a summation of parasternal short-axis planes obtained from the apex through to the base. The areas* A_1, A_2, *and* A_3 *are the planimetered areas in the parasternal short-axis projection.* L *is derived from an apical projection, usually from the apical long-axis plane.* **III.** *An expansion of method II, four parasternal short-axis slices (instead of three) are used. The longest length is the same as that used in method II. It must be noted that methods II and III make the assumption that the parasternal short-axis slices are perpendicular to the long-axis plane and equidistant from each other. We believe the assurance that this is the case cannot be substantiated.* **IV.** *Biplane area–*

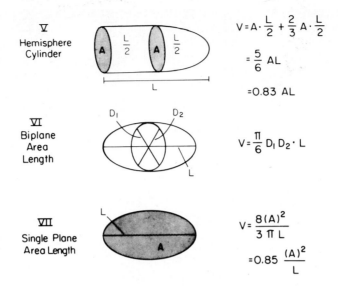

$$V = A \cdot \frac{L}{2} + \frac{2}{3} A \cdot \frac{L}{2}$$

$$= \frac{5}{6} AL$$

$$= 0.83 \ AL$$

$$V = \frac{\pi}{6} D_1 D_2 \cdot L$$

$$V = \frac{8(A)^2}{3 \pi L}$$

$$= 0.85 \ \frac{(A)^2}{L}$$

length method of the traced area outlines (A_1 and A_2) obtained from the apical long-axis and apical four-chamber planes. L is obtained from either the apical long-axis or apical four-chamber plane. This is the formula for volume of an ellipse used to calculate volume from biplane cineangiographic areas. The planes are orthogonal as shown in I. **V.** The hemisphere cylinder model uses an area obtained from the parasternal short-axis plane at the level of the papillary muscles (or the mitral valve) and a length (L) obtained from an apical long-axis plane as described in the previous method. The formulation is slightly different and is the formula for a hemisphere and cylinder. **VI.** Ellipsoid biplane technique using an apical plane, usually the long-axis apical plane, and a parasternal short-axis plane at either the level of the tips of the papillary muscles or at mitral valve level. Anteroposterior and lateral diameters (D_1 and D_2) and the length from the apical long-axis plane (L) are obtained. **VII.** Single-plane area–length method using the angiographic formula for single-plane volume analysis. This uses the planimetered area obtained from the apical long-axis or apical four-chamber view. L is the longest length.

pleted by tracing along the free wall of the ventricular endocardium and back to the cardiac apex (Fig. 15-2). The papillary muscles, when seen in this plane, are excluded from contributing to the area by drawing a line through their bases. The long axis of the ventricle is taken from the apex through the plane of the opposed mitral valve leaflets.

For the apical long-axis plane, the outline of the endocardium is traced from the apex, along the posterior wall, the opposed mitral valve leaflets, around the left ventriclar outflow area, and back to the cardiac apex. The papillary muscles, when encountered, are excluded using the technique described above. In this plane, the long axis of the left ventricle is taken from the apex through the closed mitral valve leaflets (Fig. 15-3). The end-diastolic volume and end-systolic volume are calculated based on maximum and mini-

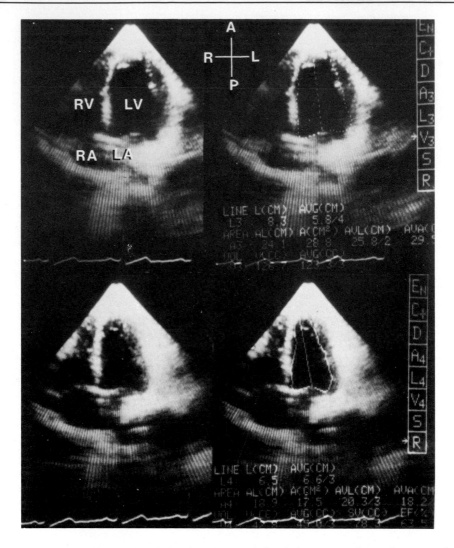

FIG. 15-2. *Demonstration of the frames used for left ventricular volume analysis from the apical four-chamber plane. The top frames were obtained at end-diastole and the bottom frames at end-systole. The right-hand figures demonstrate the endocardial outline tracing by the light pen. The left ventricle (LV) occupies the central portion of the fan. The line drawn from the opposed mitral valve leaflets through the cardiac apex represents the long axis used to derive ventricular volume. A, anterior; L, left; LA, left atrium; P, posterior; R, right; RA, right atrium: RV, right ventricle.*

mum ventricular sizes, but usually coincide with the peak of the R wave or the downslope of the T wave. The area outlines from both planes can be stored in the computer memory and the outlines subsequently recalled, and volumes calculated by single plane (Fig. 15-1, VII) and biplane area–length (Fig. 15-1, IV), and Simpson's rule methods (Fig. 15-1, I). We compared the results of the

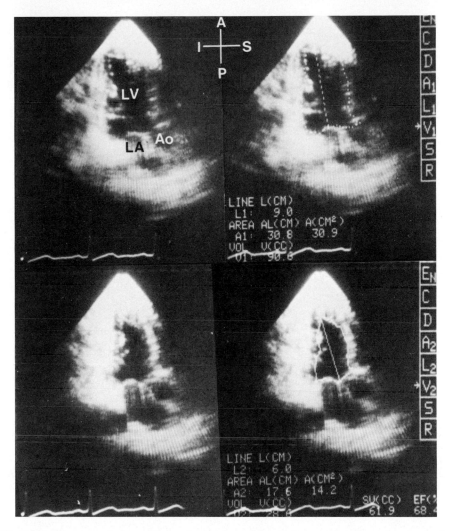

FIG. 15-3. *Demonstration of the frames used for left ventricular volume analysis from the apical long-axis plane. The left ventricle (LV) is in the central portion of the apex fan. The left atrium (LA) and aorta (Ao) are also labeled. The representation of the images and the traced outlines are identical to those shown in Fig. 15-2, end-diastolic frames on the top, end-systolic frames on the bottom. The light pen outline is shown in the right-sided panel for comparison. A, anterior; I, inferior; P, posterior; S, superior.*

angiographic estimates of left ventricular volume against these four techniques, and two additional M-mode techniques to examine the comparisons between the radiologic and echocardiographic estimates of volume (Table 15-1, Figs. 15-4 and 15-5).[14,15] We express the ejection fraction as a percent (Fig. 15-6, Table 15-1).

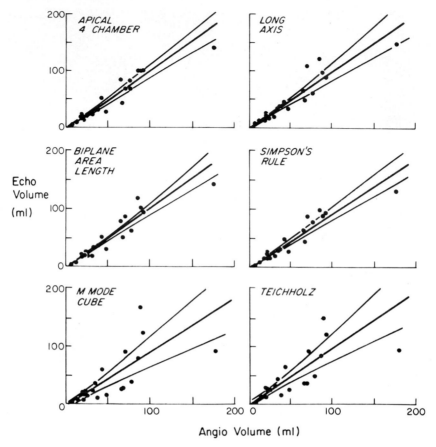

FIG. 15-4. *Comparison between the various echocardiographic methods with angiography for calculating end-diastolic volume. The four two-dimensional techniques are displayed. The top left graph shows the single-plane area–length method from the apical four-chamber plane; the top right graph shows the single-plane area–length method from the apical long-axis plane. The middle panels display the biplane methods. The middle left graph shows biplane area–length technique. The middle right graph shows a Simpson's rule method. The bottom panels contain two M-mode methods for comparison. The cube method is shown in bottom left, and the corrected cube method of Teichholz is shown in the bottom right. The angiographic volumes are displayed on the horizontal axis, and the echocardiographic variable on the vertical axis. The data points, the line of regression, and the 95 percent weighted confidence limits from the line are shown.*

We found that the calculation of end-diastolic volume by all the two-dimensional techniques correlated fairly closely to that calculated by angiography. End-systolic volumes correlated less closely with the angiographic volumes, which may be related to the inability to make the precise frame selection in infants and small children who have more rapid heart rates. Our overestimation of left ventricular and end-systolic volume by two-dimen-

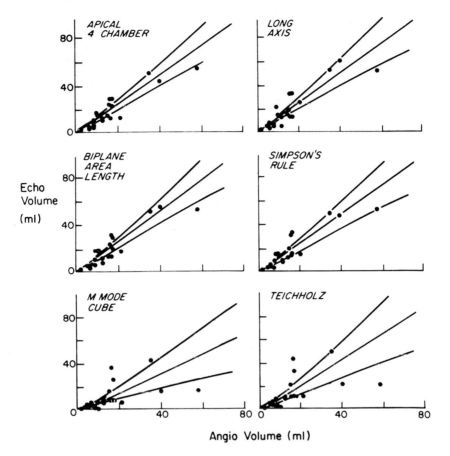

FIG. 15-5. *Comparison of the various echocardiographic methods and angiography for calculating the end-systolic volume. The regression lines, data points, confidence lines, and position of the individual comparisons is the same as for Fig. 15-4.*

sional echocardiography cannot be explained on the basis of inacurrate tracing of the endocardial echo because the endocardial echo was often easier to define at end-systole than at end-diastole. Another reason for the inaccuracy of end-systolic frame selection may be related to the inability to search as precisely for the end-systolic volume from the electrocardiogram as would be possible if a phonocardiographic trace was displayed on the video monitor. Newer systems (which use video recorders, allow slow forward and backward replay, and can display a physiologic reference such as a phonocardiogram) may allow a more precise localization of the end-systolic frame. With rapid heart rates, 30 frames per second may not be sufficient time to record the precise frame for end-systolic measurement.

Recent studies have achieved excellent estimation of ejection fraction in children using area traced from the parasternal short axis at the level of the papillary muscle (or mitral valve) from the formula $5/6 \cdot AL$, where A is the

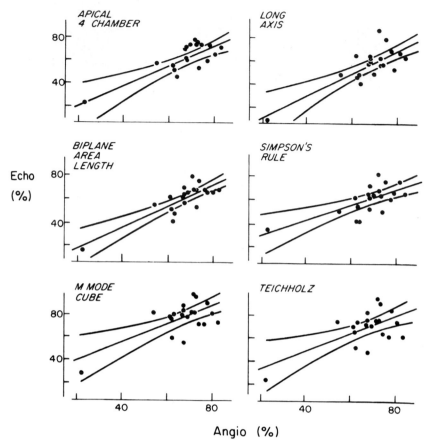

FIG. 15-6. *Comparisons of the various echocardiographic measurements and angiography for calculating the ejection fraction. The regression line, data point, and 95 percent confidence limits for the line are shown. The position of the comparisons are the same as in Figs. 15-4 and 15-5.*

cross-sectional area at the level of the papillary muscle (or at the level of the mitral valve), and L is the longest length of the ventricle from an apical view (Fig. 15-1, model V).[9,13] Single outlines of the ventricle in the parasternal short axis may not be accurate when there is incoordinate ventricular contraction. This does not appear to be a significant problem in younger children. An accurate estimation of ventricular volume can be calculated from multiple areas obtained from the parasternal short-axis plane and an apical plane to derive the long axis (Fig. 15-1, model II or III). This technique may not warrant the extra time to calculate volume because other two-dimensional techniques provide adequate estimates of volume and ejection fraction.

It has been our anecdotal experience, too, that the change in the area of the ventricle, in the parasternal short-axis plane, at papillary muscle level from end-diastole to end-systole produces a reasonable estimate of the ejec-

TABLE 15-1. LINEAR REGRESSION EQUATIONS FOR COMPARISON BETWEEN ANGIOGRAPHY (x) AND ECHOCARDIOGRAPHY (y)

Technique	Slope	Intercept	r
END-DIASTOLIC VOLUMES			
A4C	1.01	−4.15	0.97
ALA	0.98	−2.15	0.96
BAL	1.05	−3.64	0.96
SR	0.95	−3.31	0.97
Cube	0.93	−4.60	0.83
Corr Cube	0.98	−0.41	0.86
END-SYSTOLIC VOLUMES			
A4C	1.29	−1.67	0.92
ALA	1.35	−0.82	0.88
BAL	1.37*	−1.37	0.91
SR	1.25	−1.59	0.89
Cube	0.84	−1.83	0.74
Corr Cube	1.17	−1.97	0.78
EJECTION FRACTION			
A4C	0.85	+0.30	0.73
ALA	0.95	−0.80	0.77
BAL	0.87	0.00	0.82
SR	0.66*	+0.16	0.68
Cube	0.78	+0.22	0.67
Corr Cube	0.76	+0.18	0.63

* Slope significantly different from 1 at 5% level by t test.
Abbreviations: A4C, apical four-chamber method; ALA, apical long-axis method; BAL, biplane area length method; SR, Simpson's rule; Cube, M-mode cube method; Corr Cube, M-mode corrected cube method.

tion fraction when the areas are subtracted; that is, $EF = [(A_d − A_s)/A_d] \cdot 100$, where the areas planimetered, A_d and A_s, are determined at end-diastole and end-systole. The same limitation as described above on the accuracy of the formula applies when incoordinate left ventricular contraction is present.

LEFT ATRIAL VOLUME

Left atrial dimensions can be traced from several planes by both M-mode and two-dimensional echocardiography.[16,17] Left atrial area can be traced from these planes and the volumes derived from the single-plane and biplane methods (Fig. 15-7). We have compared angiographic estimates on left atrial volume against M-mode dimensionals using standard M-mode and a number of two-dimensional echocardiographic methods.[18] The two-dimensional planes we have used are the parasternal long-axis plane, and the apical four-chamber and apical long-axis planes. To achieve this, the transducer must be manipulated to produce the maximum area.

From the parasternal long-axis plane it may be necessary to place the

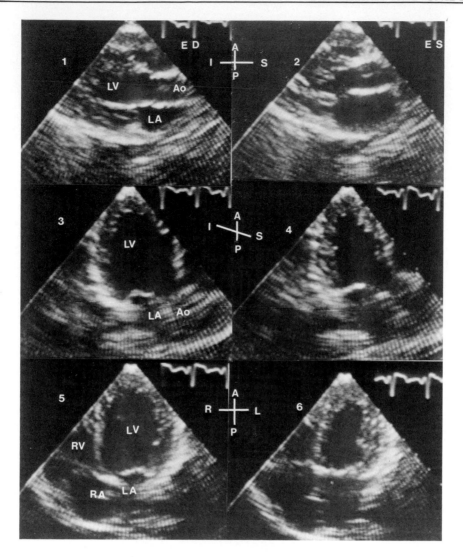

FIG. 15-7. *End-diastolic frames (ED)* **(left),** *and end-systolic frames (ES)* **(right)** *used to calculate left atrial volume. Frames* **1** *and* **2** *are parasternal long-axis views, and the parasternal view orientation is higher than usual in order to display the roof of the left atrium (LA). Frames* **3** *and* **4** *show apical long-axis views. Frames* **5** *and* **6** *show apical four-chamber views that were used to calculate the volume. Biplane measurements of left atrial volumes are possible from the combination of frames* **3** *and* **5** *for end-diastolic measurements, and frames* **4** *and* **6** *for end-systolic measurements. A, anterior; Ao, aorta; I, inferior; L, left; LV, left ventricle; P, posterior; R, right; RA, right atrium; RV, right ventricle; S, superior.*

transducer in a slightly higher interspace to image the superior extent of the left atrium. In this location the long-axis plane is obtained by placing the transducer so that the aorta occupies the center of the fan. Two apical plane scans can be obtained in the usual manner described in Chapter 3.

Care has to be taken to image the posterior left atrial wall clearly. In the apical four-chamber view the fossa ovalis is often not well imaged. In these instances a straight line is drawn over the fossa ovalis between the visible edges of the atrial septum. The origin of the pulmonary veins from the left atrium is excluded by drawing a line through the junction of the orifices of the veins with the atrium. The left atrial appendage, when identified, is excluded from the area tracing. As the mitral valve leaflets must be opposed during measurement, the line is drawn directly on the atrial surface of the mitral valve taking these points into account. Using a microcomputer system as described for left ventricular analysis, we planimetered the areas in the parasternal long-axis, apical four-chamber, and apical long-axis planes. For all three planes, the long axis (L) was represented by a line drawn between the opposed mitral valve leaflets and the posterosuperior left atrial wall. The apical long-axis and four-chamber view share a common long axis when combined for a biplane–Simpson's rule method (Fig. 15-1, I). In each plane, end-systolic and end-diastolic planes are selected for analysis. Using the peak of the R wave and the down slope of the T wave on the electrocardiogram as a guide, maximum and minimum atrial size were used as the definitive points for analysis. The comparisons with angiography for each plane are shown in Table 15-2. The correlation between all of these two-dimensional techniques with angiography is closer than with manipulation of M-mode data (Table 15-3). The best results were achieved with the apical biplane (Simpson's rule) method (Fig. 15-8, left). Single-plane–area-length techniques (Fig. 15-1, VII) yielded a reasonably good correlation with the atrial volume (Fig 15-8, right) calculated by angiography. These data are from an early study and suggest that estimation of left atrial size is possible using two-dimensional echocardiography. There is insufficient data available to judge whether the estimation of left atrial volume will be accurate enough to follow left atrial size, and this supposition awaits further study.

The left atrial size can also be evaluated from the suprasternal notch, and

TABLE 15-2. A COMPARISON OF END-SYSTOLIC AND END-DIASTOLIC PLANES WITH ANGIOGRAPHY

Algorithm	Second Echo Window and View	Regression Equation	r
Single-plane–area-length	Parasternal long-axis	$y = 0.81x + 4.5 \pm 13.8$	0.85
	Apex two-chamber	$y = 1.3x + 1.9 \pm 20.8$	0.86
	Apex four-chamber	$y = 1.2x + 8.8 \pm 26.6$	0.78
Biplane–Simpson's	Apex views paired	$y = 1.0x + 6.3 \pm 16.5$	0.86

Legend: y = volume from echocardiogram in ml, x = volume from angiogram in ml.

TABLE 15-3. A CORRELATION BETWEEN TWO-DIMENSIONAL TECHNIQUES AND M-MODE DATA

M-Mode–Echo Dimension	Regression Equation	r
A-P diameter in mm.	$y = 1.5x - 10.9$	0.50
(A-P diameter)^3	$y = 0.68x - 13.4$	0.46
A-P diameter as power function	$y = 3.7x^{1.8}$	0.69

Legend: y and x are same as in Table 15-2, except for the last equation where y = angiographic volume and x = echocardiographic volume.

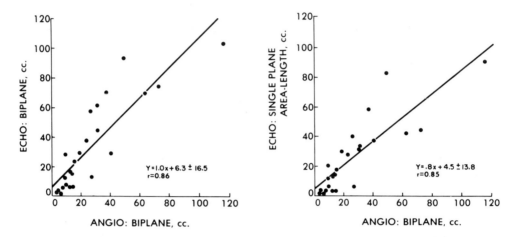

FIG. 15-8. *Graphic display of the best echocardiographic correlations of left atrial volume with angiography as shown in Table 15-2. The data were obtained in 12 patients with body surface areas of 0.37 to 2.01 M². Covariance analysis showed the volumes could be displayed as a single linear function.* **Left.** *The apical left atrial outlines were combined using a Simpson's rule method (Fig. 15-1, I).* **Right.** *The best single-plane estimate of left atrial volume was achieved with a single-plane area–length method from the parasternal long-axis plane (Fig. 15-1, VII). The data points, regression line, correlation coefficients, and standard errors of the estimate are shown for each comparison.*

from parasternal and subcostal planes. The combination of any of these views for calculating left atrial volume has not been attempted using two-dimensional echocardiography.

RIGHT-SIDED MEASUREMENTS

Because of the irregular geometry of the right ventricle, it is difficult to develop a formula for calculating right ventricular volume by two-dimensional echocardiography. It has also been difficult to image the entire right ventric-

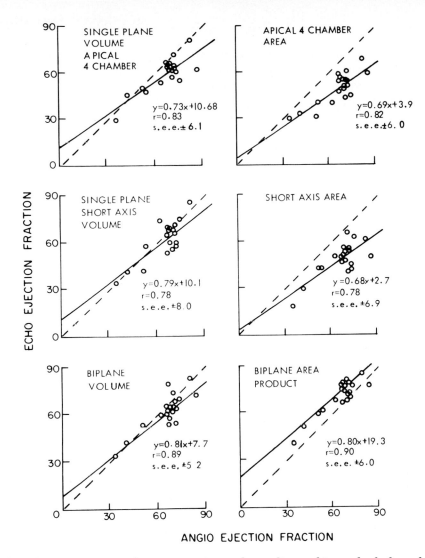

FIG. 15-9. *Comparisons between various echocardiographic methods for calculating right ventricular ejection fraction on the vertical axis (echo) and ejection fraction derived from biplane right ventricular angiography (angio) on the horizontal axis. The regression line is shown as a continuous line, the line of identity as a dashed line, and the data points as open circles, N = 20. The regression equation, correlation coefficient, and standard error of the estimate (s.e.e.) are shown for each comparison. The left-sided figures demonstrate a comparison between angiographic ejection fraction and ejection fraction derived from volume calculations. The top left graph shows ejection fraction calculated from the apical four-chamber area–length volume. The middle left graph shows the ejection fraction from the parasternal short-axis area–length volume. The bottom left is a biplane method using a combination of areas with a length (see text for detail). The right-sided figures demonstrate a comparison between ejection fraction by angiography and a percent change in the areas. The top right is the percent area change from the apical four-chamber plane. The middle right shows percent change using the short-axis area, and the bottom right shows a percent change of the products of the areas from these two planes from end-diastole to end-systole (see text for detail). These 20 patients ranged in age from 1 month to 10 years and had body surface areas of 0.25 to 1.14 M².*

ular outline in any one view except in the apical four-chamber plane. Because of the inability to obtain a common long axis from a combination of views and the geometrical shape, the use of biplane measurements from two or more right ventricular planes to estimate ventricular volumes has been difficult. The work to date for calculating right ventricular size and function in children and adults has used only the apical four-chamber view to evaluate right ventricular size. While it is still preliminary, the correlation of increasing or decreasing right ventricular size by two-dimensional echocardiography with angiography appears to be superior to that which can be obtained by M-mode echocardiography.[12,19,20]

We have explored a combination of apical four-chamber right ventricular areas and those obtained from the parasternal short-axis plane where the area is maximized. Volumes from each plane were determined at end-diastole and end-systole using a single-plane area–length algorithm and from the biplane formula: $V = 0.849 \, (A_{SA} \cdot A_{A4C})/L$, where A equals the area in the short axis (SA) and apical four-chamber planes (A4C), and L is the longest length of the ventricle obtained from the apical four-chamber plan (Fig. 15-9).[21]

Our preliminary findings support published observations. There is an underestimation in the volume calculated by these two-dimensional techniques. However, the underestimation was proportioned in both systole and diastole so that a reasonable estimate of the ejection fraction from the right ventricle can be obtained (Fig. 15-8). We explored several algorithms in addition to those mentioned above. Reasonable correlations with the area for ejection fraction were obtained when calculating the area changes that occur from diastole (A_d) and systole (A_s), where the ejection fraction $EF = [(A_d - A_s)/A_d] \cdot 100$. We used a product of the areas in diastole from the four-chamber and parasternal short-axis planes to evaluate whether the ejection fraction could be calculated reliably from the formula $[(Pr_D - Pr_S)/Pr_D] \cdot 100$, when $Pr =$ product $A_{A4C} \cdot A_{SA}$, D and S are end-diastole, and end-systole.

A close linear correlation was obtained with this technique and compares favorably with the biplane volume measurement (Fig. 15-9). Several manipulations of the area measurements in different planes are possible but to date we have found short-axis and apical four-chamber measurement to be the most regularly achievable planes.

THE RIGHT ATRIAL SIZE

There have been only two attempts to estimate right atrial size by two-dimensional echocardiography. These studies measured either the area of the right atrium planimetered from the apical four-chamber plane[12] or measured its anteroposterior or superoinferior dimensions.[19] Increase or decrease of right atrial size can be compared with the expected normal size for body surface area.

At present, the calculation of chamber volume is time consuming, and in our laboratory the tracing of a single frame takes the same amount of time as it

CHAPTER 16

Photographic Techniques

The reproduction of still-frame images is an important aspect of the technique of two-dimensional echocardiography. The still-frame image is an essential communication medium for publications, teaching, and other presentations. Because there are thirty frames generated every second, there are times during the cardiac cycle when an ideal single frame is available for photography. In patients with rapid heart rates, the opportunity to photograph a still-frame image may be limited by the rapid motion of the cardiac valves and walls. Stop-frame images without blurring occur when there is minimal cardiac motion, such as at end-diastole or end-systole. In addition, atrioventricular valves can be photographed without motion artifact in diastole between the V and A waves.

The well-reproduced, still-frame image requires attention to detail from its actual generation to the making of the final print. Unless the ultrasound equipment is satisfactory, a good picture cannot be reproduced. For the purposes of this chapter we must assume that adequate images have been obtained by the ultrasound equipment. The technique of photography described below was used to make the photographs for this volume.

THE SCREEN

We prefer a black-and-white television monitor for generating photographs. The ease with which the contrast and brightness can be controlled makes it superior to standard green oscilloscopes or low persistence phosphors. We have not used frame-freeze or multiple-cycle, ECG-triggered images for photography because they are time consuming and contain no more data than are available in a good frame-freeze image from the video recorder.

The video monitor should be of the highest quality because poorer quality monitors produce poorer quality pictures. The brightness and contrast controls should be adjusted to produce a visually satisfactory picture (Fig. 16-1). Contrast or brightness levels that are too low (Fig. 16-2) or too high (Fig. 16-3) detract from the quality of the photographic reproduction.

THE CAMERA

Most ultrasound systems use some form of a Polaroid camera, although newer systems with digital scan converters can reproduce images on the same silver iodide paper used to make black-and-white M-mode echocardiographic recordings.

Some ultrasound systems use an automatic Polaroid camera system in which the contrast and brightness controls of the video screen can be varied while the shutter speed and the lens aperture cannot be altered easily. This system is not ideal for making photographs because the operator cannot control the important factors involved in generating a well-exposed image.

We use a Polaroid CU 5 camera with an 8 × 10 inch hood and lens (Fig. 16-4). Various size hoods are available for different size television screens. The lens is in focus when the hood makes contact with the television screen. The camera has a trigger shutter release, variable shutter speed, and lens aperture (f stop) control. We use a 13-inch video screen that is slightly larger than the hood. This slight mismatch allows some magnification of the image so that more of the film can be filled with the image. The image cannot be magnified further without visualization of the raster lines on the video monitor.

FILM TYPE

Several film types are available for Polaroid cameras (Fig. 16-1, Table 16-1). Polaroid 084 film, the standard black-and-white film available for Polaroid cameras, was the first type of film used. This film is a rapidly developing, panchromatic film that requires application of protective coating after the film has developed. The film has medium contrast and is extremely light sensitive (ASA 3000). For producing an adequate image, the shutter speed should be 1/15 of a second with a lens aperture of between $f11$ and $f16$.

More recently, films that do not require coating have been developed. The Polaroid 667 film, which is a modification of the 084 film, is a medium-contrast panchromatic film that requires 30 seconds to develop adequately. The film must be removed from contact with the developing paste after 30 seconds or else the developing process will continue. The 667 film requires a shutter speed of 1/15 of a second with a lens aperture of between $f11$ and $f16$.

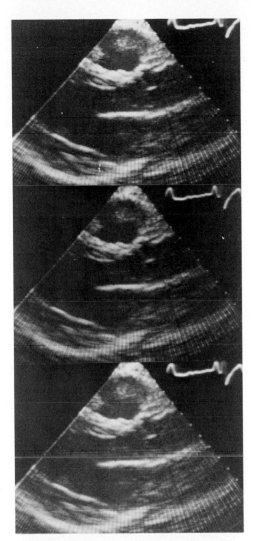

FIG. 16-1. *Three photographs of the same still-frame image taken from a television screen using three different Polaroid films. The contrast and brightness settings on the television monitor were the same for all three photographs.* **Top.** *084 film exposed for 1/15 of a second at f11.* **Middle.** *667 film exposed for 1/15 of a second at f11.* **Bottom.** *611 film exposed for 1/4 of a second at f11. The final photographs were reproduced on professional copy film (Kodak 4125).*

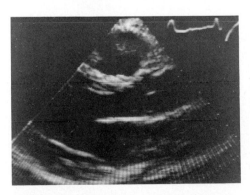 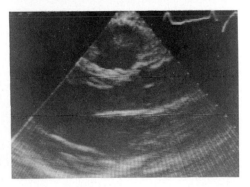

FIG. 16-2. **Left.** *A photograph taken from a video monitor in which the contrast setting was satisfactory but the brightness setting was too low.* **Right.** *A photograph taken from a videomonitor in which the brightness setting was at a normal level but the contrast setting was too low.*

267

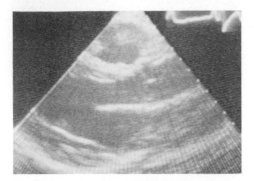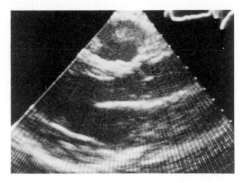

FIG. 16-3. *These photographs were taken from a video monitor with excessive brightness and contrast settings.* **Left.** *A photograph taken from a video monitor with too much brightness and normal contrast.* **Right.** *A photograph taken from a video monitor with too much contrast and normal brightness.*

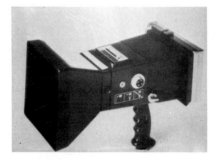

FIG. 16-4. *A photograph of a Polaroid CU 5 camera used for production of the illustrations in this volume. The camera has a hand-held unit with a trigger-released shutter control and a hood that can be changed depending on the size of the television screen.*

Polaroid 611 film, the most recent development in instant films, was used to produce most of the illustrations in this volume. Polaroid 611 film is a panchromatic film with low contrast and relatively less light sensitivity than the 084 and 667 films. The 611 film requires a shutter speed of 1/4 of a second with a lens aperture of between $f11$ to $f16$. It has better gray-scale characteristics than the other films described above and is recommended by the Polaroid corporation as the film of choice for two-dimensional echocardiography. Although we used Polaroid 611 film for most of the illustrations in this volume, we found that almost any type of film produces satisfactory images for reproduction (Fig. 16-1). We prefer instant developing film to images developed on silver iodide paper from digital scan converters because of the greater sensitivity of the former technique. Satisfactory photographs can be made with a 35-mm camera and film; however, this technique is less desirable because

TABLE 16-1. POLAROID FILM

	084	667	611
ASA speed	3000	3000	200
Contrast	medium	medium	low
Resolution (line pairs/mm)	16–22	16–20	20
Coating	yes	no	no
Continuous development after film removed from the camera	no	yes	no
Processing time @ 20° C	15 sec	45 sec	45 sec
Shutter speed	1/15	1/15	1/4
Aperture	f11–f16	f11–f16	f11–f16
Comments	Coating messy	Continuous development unsatisfactory	Low contrast and slower ASA rating make this a film of choice

one has to wait for the developing and printing to see whether the photographs are satisfactory.

Once a satisfactory print has been obtained, it is cropped, labeled, and sent to the photographer for reproduction. The photographer used professional copy film (Kodak 4125) and medium-contrast paper (usually Kodak RC2 or RC3 paper) for reproduction of almost all of the pictures in this volume. The photographer used a 4 × 5 inch camera because the negative is easier to manipulate than 35-mm film; however, we have used 35-mm film with excellent results.

Almost as much variation can be introduced into the reproduction of the copied film as in the original Polaroid print. The photographic department should reproduce the original print using continuous tone rather than high-contrast or lithographic film. Lithographic film or high-contrast film artificially enhances some of the characteristics of the original but removes the gray scale shading from the film, thereby diminishing the quality of the reproduction (Fig. 16-5). The resulting photograph is similar to that produced by having excessive contrast on the television monitor.

In reproducing the final print, changes in the contrast grade of the paper or the degree of exposure may cause quite significant changes in the reproduction. These changes can be used to improve substandard originals (Figs. 16-6 and 16-7). A good photographer can produce a good picture from original photographs of variable quality (Fig. 16-8); however, the best results are obtained when an adequate print is presented to the photographer. In this way the final print can be made that corresponds to the original in tone and contrast characteristics. The final prints were designed to be 3 inches wide (column width) when reproduced. In this way, the final print saves space, can be reproduced without reduction by the printer, and is suitable for most journals with columns.

We make our own slides from either the final print or from the original

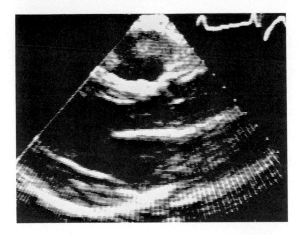

FIG. 16-5. *The original photograph shown on the bottom of Fig. 16-1 reproduced with lithographic (high-contrast film). The effect of using this high-contrast film is similar to the effect produced by having excessive contrast on the video monitor (Fig. 16-3, right).*

FIG. 16-6. *This photograph was produced from the right panel of Fig. 16-2 using Kodabrome II RC-UH to enhance the contrast. Note that the quality of the reproduction approaches the quality of Fig. 16-1 (bottom).*

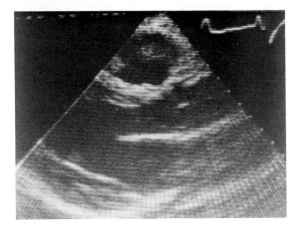

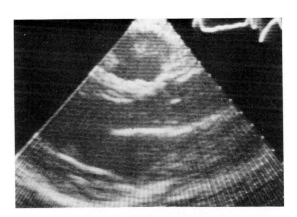

FIG. 16-7. *This photograph was produced from the left panel of Fig. 16-3 using an ultra-hard Kodabrome paper and an adjusted exposure. The quality of this reproduction approaches the quality of Fig. 16-1 (bottom).*

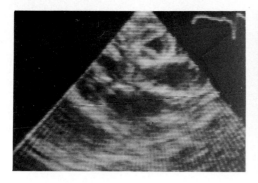 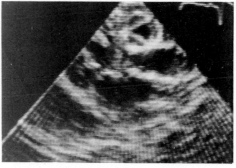

FIG. 16-8. *The left frame is the original Polaroid photograph obtained to show the pulmonary valve. The right frame was obtained by reproducing the left frame on a special paper to enhance the contrast.*

Polaroid before and/or after labeling. We use a standard 35-mm, single-lens reflex camera (with a close-up lens) mounted on a Polaroid copy stand with four 150-watt reflector bulbs. Recently we have changed the lighting by using two 600-watt Glenwood Halogen Lamps (3400 K—Griffith, Indiana). We use Kodak SO 185 film* that we develop in the hospital's automatic x-ray processor. This film can be fed into the developer using the safety lights. Exposure of this film depends on the intensity of the lighting. For our own lighting system (which can only be used as a guide), the exposure times are approximately 7 seconds with an aperture of *f*4. The film is extremely slow with an ASA rating of less than 1 (compared to Polaroid 084, with a rating of 3000 ASA). The slide film is extremely economical. We estimate that the final cost of printing a slide, including the process of mounting, is less than five cents.

* Now called Kodak Rapid Process Copy film.

Index